The Comp
Home Remedies
for Your Cat

**Look for this other pet-care title
by Deborah Mitchell**

*The Complete Book of
Home Remedies for Your Dog*

Now available from St. Martin's Paperbacks

The Complete Book of
Home Remedies
for Your Cat

Deborah Mitchell

A Lynn Sonberg Book

St. Martin's Paperbacks

The information in this book is not intended to replace the advice of a veterinarian, who should be consulted in matters relating to your pet's health, especially if your pet has existing medical conditions. Individual readers are solely responsible for their own decisions related to their pet's health. The author and the publisher do not accept responsibility for any adverse effects individuals may claim that their pet experiences, whether directly or indirectly, from the information contained in this book.

The fact that an organization or web site is mentioned in the book as a potential source of information does not mean that the author or publisher endorse any of the information they may provide or recommendations they may make.

THE COMPLETE BOOK OF HOME REMEDIES FOR YOUR CAT

Copyright © 2013 by Lynn Sonberg Book Associates.

All rights reserved.

For information address St. Martin's Press, 175 Fifth Avenue, New York, NY 10010.

EAN: 978-1-250-02628-6

Printed in the United States of America

St. Martin's Paperbacks edition / May 2013

St. Martin's Paperbacks are published by St. Martin's Press, 175 Fifth Avenue, New York, NY 10010.

10 9 8 7 6 5 4 3 2 1

Contents

Introduction

Welcome fellow cat lovers! As you know, when you accept a cat into your household—or should I say, when cats allow you to share their space with them!—it's like welcoming a new member to the family. While cats can be annoyingly aloof and independent creatures, they also need lots of love, nurturing, and attention, especially when it comes to feeding and health care. Even the most independent cat needs a responsible health care advocate and pet parent rolled into one, and that person is probably you and your family.

WHY HOME REMEDIES FOR CATS?

It makes sense: If you are among the growing number of people who is taking more control of their own nutritional needs and health care choices, often those choices include natural and home remedies. Those same types of options are available for your cat.

For example, Sarah realized that taking care of Tuxedo's teeth was important, and that failing to do so regularly could prove costly both in terms of money and her cat's health. So she learned how to clean Tuxedo's teeth at home and uses an herb (plantain) to control tartar and support gum health. Now, whenever she takes Tuxedo to his veterinarian, the doctor is amazed at how healthy the cat's teeth and gums are.

When Karl's Siamese mix, Sophia, got ear mites, he didn't want to rely on conventional medications, so he turned to a home remedy that included olive oil for the ears and a homemade shampoo consisting of hydrogen peroxide, borax, vitamin E, and water to safely eliminate those pests without using harsh chemicals.

Why should you consider home remedies for your cat? Not surprisingly, the reasons to use them to support healthy living are much the same for your pet, yourself and your family. For example:

- **Peace of mind.** Having an understanding of which home remedies can provide symptom relief can help you feel more confident you'll be able to care for your cat when the need arises, such as an acute case of hair balls, or knowing which home remedies can help take care of your cat's dental problems or help her drop a few pounds.
- **Saving money.** Home remedies are often less expensive than prescriptions or visits to the veterinarian. In fact, some remedies cost only pennies. For example, you can use apple cider vinegar for allergic dermatitis, olive oil for ear mites, and pumpkin seeds for intestinal worms. Use of home remedies can also allow you to significantly reduce the need for any prescription medication your veterinarian may prescribe.
- **More control.** Home remedies give you more of a sense of control over your cat's well-being.
- **Minimizing or eliminating side effects.** Natural home remedies can reduce or eliminate your cat's exposure to medication or other treatments that may cause side effects that can significantly affect your cat's quality of life.

The home remedies offered in this book—from the dietary suggestions to the nutritional supplements, herbal remedies, and more—help promote and support the body's ability to heal itself or regain its natural balance. In some cases the remedies may be used along with conventional treatments offered by your veterinarian. This integrative approach is a more harmonious way to support the body's healing process.

YOU ARE YOUR CAT'S HEALTH ADVOCATE

A cat's independent streak doesn't extend to important tasks such as buying her own food, ridding herself of ear mites, getting insulin injections, or driving herself to the veterinarian. These tasks and more are your responsibility as your cat's health advocate.

It is becoming easier to find veterinarians who have adopted a holistic approach to caring for their patients, with a more focused effort on dietary and nutritional needs (including homemade foods for your cat) and techniques beyond traditional vaccinations and medications, such as herbal remedies, acupuncture, and nutritional supplements. Similarly, an increasing number of pet parents (the term I use throughout the book rather than "pet owner") are receptive to and want to learn more about home remedies for their cats.

A key component of home remedies for cats is diet and nutrition. Although the immune system in cats and people is designed to promote balance and self-healing, you can throw a big monkey wrench into the works if you don't provide your cat with balanced nutrition based on his inherent needs as well as his age and health status. Poor nutrition can severely compromise a cat's immune system and overall health, sometimes rapidly, especially when your cat suffers an injury, infection, or disease.

Your role as pet parent and health advocate is to ensure your kitty has the nutrition necessary to support and maintain health, to offer home remedies that can take care of situations that can be handled with love and care at home, and to know when to seek help from a professional veterinarian or feline nutritionist.

HOW TO USE THIS BOOK

This book is divided into two parts. The first part is "Feline Cuisine and Nutrition," and it's first because optimal nutrition is the cornerstone of your cat's health and well-being. If you learn how to provide your cat with foods that support and promote his immune system, you will have a solid basis for his overall health and a strong ally in the fight against illness and disease.

How much do you know about cat food? Part of your responsibility as your cat's health advocate is understanding her nutritional needs and which foods can meet those needs. If you depend on what you read on the bag or can of cat food or what you hear or read about in ads for cat food, then you may be sadly misinformed. Your cat does not care if the cat food can is a pretty color, if his dry food is shaped like a fish, or if his food is served in a crystal stemmed glass: That's all marketing for your sake.

You may have heard someone say at one time or another, "I wouldn't feed that to my cat." The trouble is, much of the commercial cat food on the market *shouldn't* be fed to your cat. That's why the three opening chapters in the book in part I focus on the nutrition your cat needs, which foods can provide that nutrition, and how to make your own homemade cat food—including recipes—to ensure your cat is getting what she needs to thrive.

I can appreciate that not everyone has the time nor the inclination to scour over cat food labels and/or prepare homemade food for their cat. For those readers who do, these first three chapters provide lots of detailed information on cat food ingredients. For other readers, this book also provides suggestions on some of the highest-quality commercial cat foods on the market so they can be sure to give their kitties the very best.

Part II is titled "Feline Conditions and Home Remedies;" it's where you can find detailed information about the most common ailments and diseases that affect cats, including symptoms, which breeds are more susceptible to the complaint, and how the problem is typically treated. Each entry also explains which home remedies may help and how you can work with your veterinarian or on your own to apply them.

One downfall when it comes to the use of natural supplements and home remedies for cats is a shortage of double-blind, placebo-controlled studies to back up their use. However, there is no shortage of anecdotal reports from pet parents and years of clinical experience from veterinary professionals who have years of personal, clinical experience with their feline clients. In addition, an increased interest in natural treatment options from veterinary schools and research facilities is opening the doors to more choices for our feline family members.

Veterinarians generally agree that to be a good cat health advocate, you should provide your cat with a nutritious diet, see that she has physical and mental stimulation, take her for yearly checkups, adhere to the recommended vaccination schedules, and use preventive tick and flea methods. If you are among the many pet parents who don't always meet all of these recommended goals, you are not alone. However, that does not mean you don't want to provide the best you can for your cat. This book can serve as a tool to help you be a better health advocate for your cat when it comes to nutrition, managing common health challenges when they arise, and providing home remedies that meet those needs.

PART I

Feline Cuisine and Nutrition

What picture comes to mind when you first hear the words "feline cuisine"? A Sphinx-like cat holding court over a bowl (crystal, of course) heaped high with canned cat food? Your cat looking disdainfully at you with narrowed eyes as you set a bowl of kibble before her? Endless selections of canned, semimoist, and bagged cat good choices as far as the eye can see?

Feeding your cat can be as easy as opening a can once or twice a day or filling his bowl with dry food: Fill it and forget it. After all, that's one reason why there's commercial cat food so readily available, promising to deliver all the nutrition your cat needs.

The three chapters in this section on feline cuisine cover nutritional information, tips, and recipes that are a critical part of the foundation of your cat's health. The dietary and nutritional suggestions support the home remedies offered in the later chapters that will help promote and maintain your cat's health and assist in preventing or minimizing health challenges that may come her way.

Chapter 1, "Basic Nutrition: What Your Cat Needs," explores the details of a cat's nutritional requirements and contains a critical section, "How Much Food Does My Cat Need?" If you decide to skip chapter 1, at least check out this section. Chapter 2, "Cat Food: You Expect Me to Eat This?" explains how to read and analyze cat food labels. Some readers will find the information in these first two chapters of great interest (and perhaps a little disturbing at times!), but if you just want the bottom line on commercial cat foods, you can turn to page 41 in chapter 2 to read about recommended high-quality commercial cat foods that can meet your cat's needs. For cat parents who want to enter the exciting world of homemade cat food, chapter 3, "What's for Dinner? Good Food for Your Cat" is for you.

Chapter 1
Basic Nutrition: What Your Cat Needs

These scenes may be familiar: your beloved Simon was "fine" until one day you woke up and he couldn't pee, and you had to rush him to the veterinary clinic. Or Samantha was "fine" until one day she stopped eating; then she began to lose weight, and when you got her to the veterinarian, he announced she had diabetes. Or Marco was "fine" until he began scratching so much he was drawing blood and risking infection.

What do all of these scenarios have in common? An underlying cause of the problem in each case could be diet. Let's face it: cat food makers have done a good marketing job of convincing the public that everything their cats need can be found in a bag of kibble or in a can with a picture of an adorable cat on the label. You may have a pretty good idea how much vitamin C you and your family need or how much protein you should get per day, but can you say the same for your cat?

Your cat depends on you to provide her with the nutrients and overall diet she needs, and that includes knowing how much and which kinds of protein, carbohydrates, fats, and different nutrients are necessary to safeguard her from illness and disease and keep her content and functioning at her very best. So before you dish out her next meal, take a little time to learn what should be in the food on your cat's menu—and what shouldn't be.

NUTRIENTS EVERY CAT NEEDS

You and your family can turn to the U.S. Department of Health and Human Services or to the U.S. Department of Agriculture and the new "food plate" if you want to know the RDA—recommended daily allowance—of certain nutrients for your health; you can also read the nutritional information on every package of food you buy. But where do you turn if you want information on the nutrients your cat needs? Who is responsible for making sure the food on the market for your cat is safe and nutritious?

The National Academy of Sciences has set standards for specific nutritional requirements for cats. In addition, the Food and Drug Administration (FDA) regulates pet food, requiring that it be "safe to eat, produced under sanitary conditions, contain no harmful substances, and be truthfully labeled." Standards for cat food manufacturers have been established by the Association of American Feed Control Officials (AAFCO). Because the topic of commercial cat food is complex, a fuller discussion of this topic is found in chapter 2.

Every cat needs certain amounts of macronutrients (protein, carbohydrates, fats), micronutrients (vitamins, minerals, enzymes), and water not only to survive but for optimal health. However, while each cat is unique, and therefore has nutritional needs that depend on her age, size, breed, presence of any health problems, body weight, whether she is taking medications, and other factors, there are still basic nutrients that all cats need.

Let's look at the macronutrients your cat needs and a critically important message about carbohydrates before we move on to water and nutritional elements.

Protein

Cats are protein-guzzlers: they need *lots* of protein, even more than dogs do. It appears cats metabolize proteins differently than dogs do, which increases their need for protein. They are therefore inherently geared to break down large quantities of protein to glucose, from which they get their energy. Protein is also essential for your cat's growth and development, as well as optimal functioning of the immune system and all bodily functions.

If your cat were still living in the wild, then his diet would naturally consist of about 50 to 60 percent protein, 30 to 50 percent fat, and 5 to 10 percent carbohydrates. Since Jasper is domesticated and doesn't need to hunt for his food or expend the energy to do so, his protein needs have been downgraded somewhat. According to AAFCO, which sets pet food standards and is discussed in depth later, today's domesticated adult cats need only 26 percent protein, although many veterinarians and other animal experts say 35 to 50 percent or more is preferred.

Not all protein is created equal, and each source of protein contains different amounts of amino acids and differs in how your cat's body can utilize them. The ability of a protein source to be used by the body and the amount of usable amino acids is called the biological value. The food with the highest biological value is the egg, which is assigned a value of 100. Next best are fish meal and milk (92), followed by beef (about 78); soybean meal (67); meat meal, bone meal, and wheat (about 50); and corn (45).

Cats need twenty-two amino acids to make the protein necessary for their optimal health, and they can synthesize only eleven of them. That means they must get the remaining eleven from their diet. Those remaining eleven include arginine, histidine, isoleucine, leucine, lysine, methionine, phenylalanine, taurine, threonine, tryptophan, and valine.

Both taurine and arginine deserve special mention. Cats need a high amount of taurine for eye and heart health and to form bile, yet they have limited enzyme ability to produce the amino acid. Therefore, they need lots of taurine in their diet or they can develop a heart condition called dilated cardiomyopathy, undergo retinal degeneration, and have reproductive problems. If you've ever heard the warning that cats should not eat dog food, it's because dog food does not contain taurine, since they can make enough of their own.

Arginine is an important amino acid because it binds ammonia that is produced when protein is metabolized. Cats who do not get enough arginine can experience excessive salivation and vocalization and even death if ammonia levels get too high. While most animals can make arginine using the amino acid ornithine through various processes, cats make ornithine only one way: by converting arginine. Therefore, cats who don't have enough arginine can't make enough ornithine.

Cats can get their protein from either animal or plant sources, although most experts agree the preferred source is animal. (Cats can be vegetarians if their pet parents follow a rigid dietary plan and ensure their cats get taurine from supplemental sources, since it is found naturally in meat and eggs only.)

Carbohydrates

You were probably taught that carbohydrates are the body's main source of energy, but a cat's biological makeup is not geared to most efficiently metabolize carbohydrates for energy. Instead, cats get the majority of their energy from the glucose they glean from protein. Thus, cats require a small amount of carbohydrates, approximately 5 to 10 percent of their daily caloric intake.

However, if you read the ingredient label of many cat food products, especially dry foods, you will see a high percentage of ingredients that provide carbohydrates, such as ground corn, wheat flour, soybean meal, corn gluten meal, and brewer's rice, and typically these items are among the top three ingredients.

Here is a critical message about cats and carbohydrates, and it is one that you will see throughout the book: **Cats are not designed by nature to consume a lot of carbohydrates, and a high-carbohydrate diet (e.g., dry cat food) contributes to a wealth of health problems in cats.** Therefore, the best home remedies you can give your cat every day of her life are high-protein, moderate-fat, and very low-carbohydrate meals, either those you prepare yourself (recipes are provided in this book), through high-quality canned or fresh foods, or a combination of both.

If you are asking yourself, "But why are there so many

dry cat foods on the market?" "Why hasn't my veterinarian recommended I switch to canned or homemade food?"* and "How do I know which foods are best to feed my cat?" those and other questions are answered in this book.

For now, however, let's look at the results of a recent study published in the *Journal of Experimental Biology,* in which investigators conducted an extensive analysis of macronutrients in domesticated adult cats. Briefly, they set out to determine if these cats, when given a choice, would choose foods that are naturally and biologically appropriate for them, as they would in the wild. Or, as I like to put it: would they would pick the fast-food cheeseburger and fries or the grilled chicken and shrimp.

The researchers discovered that, when given a choice, the cats chose high-protein foods every single time instead of high-carbohydrate foods, even when they were provided with less of the high-protein food. They also found that when the cats were offered only high-carbohydrate foods (like dry cat food), they did not consume enough of it to meet their necessary daily need for protein.

Biologically this all makes sense, because cats don't have the enzymes necessary to digest carbohydrates. In addition, cats have low absorption rates for glucose in their intestinal tract and no taste receptors for sugar.

In other words, pet parents, cats are not made to eat carbs. If you significantly limit the carbohydrates in the food you feed your cat and provide the high-protein, moderate fat content they need, you will end up with a healthier, happier cat.

Fats

Cats need fats as an energy source and to help them absorb fat-soluble vitamins, such as vitamins A, D, E, and K. However, the fats cats need and what they get from most commercial cat foods—especially dry food—are often not the same.

---

* More and more veterinarians are.

One problem is that storing foods at high heat and/or humidity can cause fats to turn rancid and breaks down fatty acids. Another problem is many commercial cat foods contain too much fat, which is one contributing factor to the high prevalence of obesity among cats (see chapter 16, "Obesity"). A healthy range of fat for your cat is 30 to 40 percent of caloric intake.

Cats require the essential fatty acids linoleic, alpha-linolenic, and arachidonic acid in their diet, and the latter especially must come from food because cats are unable to synthesize it. Arachidonic acid is found in animal fats and is necessary for proper blood clotting, functioning of the gastrointestinal and reproductive systems, and skin growth. Arachidonic acid is a good-guy/bad-guy fatty acid because it is also necessary to produce an inflammatory response like the one that occurs in allergies. Sometimes, however, an inflammatory response is necessary because it helps the body protect itself.

The bottom line is cats need arachidonic acid in their diet, but not too much. Overall, essential fatty acids should make up at least 2 percent of your cat's daily caloric intake to prevent deficiencies. The richest sources of linoleic acid are safflower and corn oils, while fish oil is an excellent source of arachidonic acid.

MORE NUTRIENTS EVERY CAT NEEDS

Water

Water needs to be mentioned separately because cats do not have a strong drive to drink water the way many other species do. Perhaps the saying should be "You can lead a cat to water but you can't make him drink." Therefore, if you feed your cat a dry food diet, it is very possible he is not getting enough water, even if she drinks water from a bowl. Thus, cats be in a chronic state of dehydration if dry kibble is the main or only source of their diet. Canned foods and homemade foods contain much more water and therefore provide water levels that are close to what cats require for optimal health.

The take-home message: dump the dry food and switch to homemade food or at least high-quality canned foods for your cat. Bladder and urinary tract problems are common in cats, and the main reasons this is true are the lack of sufficient water in a cat's diet and the associated use of dry cat food.

Fiber

Fiber consists of various compounds found in plants, and all of them are classified as carbohydrates. Two main forms of fiber exist in nature, although all sources of fiber contain some of each form in varying percentages:

- **Insoluble, which mean it does not dissolve in water.** Insoluble fiber gives plants their structure, and it is especially helpful in helping move food through the intestinal tract. Foods that contain a high percentage of insoluble fiber include brown rice, carrots, root vegetables, and wheat bran.
- **Soluble, which means it does dissolve in water.** Good sources of soluble fiber include barley, beans, fruits, oats, peas, and vegetables.

Since cats don't need much carbohydrates, they also don't need much fiber. That said, a little fiber can go a long way in a cat's life. Small amounts of fiber help enhance intestinal health, and some health problems (e.g., constipation and diarrhea) can be helped by the addition of fiber. In commercial cat food, fiber is usually in the form of hulls (peanut, rice, and soybean), beet pulp, pectin, and bran. Homemade cat food typically includes fiber in the form of a small amount of mashed beans or cooked vegetables.

It was widely believed for many years that a diet high in fiber was good for cats who have diabetes to control blood sugar levels. However, that approach has now been found to be ill-advised (see chapter 8, "Diabetes").

Vitamins

Cats have specific requirements for nearly every vitamin except one: vitamin C, which kitties are able to produce themselves. Vitamin C is important for healing and for enhancing immune system functioning. Supplements of vitamin C could be helpful in treating urinary tract infections (see chapter 17, "Urinary Tract Infections").

Here is what you need to know about your cat's requirements for the other vitamins. The amounts are the minimums set by the AAFCO and are based on the amount of food consumed on a dry-matter basis.

- **Vitamin A.** The yellow pigment (carotene) in plants is the main source of vitamin A. While dogs can easily convert carotene into usable vitamin A, cats do not have the enzyme necessary for this conversion. Therefore, cats must get vitamin A in a form known as retinyl palmitate. This is important for pet parents to know because when looking at food and supplements labels, you want to be sure to get the correct form of vitamin A. Cats need 5,000 IU/kg while kittens need 9,000 IU/kg vitamin A daily.
- **Vitamin B complex.** The B family of vitamins are found in meat, poultry, fish, organ meats, and vegetables and are important for growth and for nerve support, function, and regeneration. All the B vitamins are water soluble, which means they are not retained by the body and are typically eliminated in the urine. B vitamins help with blood circulation and red blood cell formation, energy, adrenal function, brain function, and the health of the immune system. Because the B vitamins work synergistically, they should be taken as a combination (B complex) if you use a supplement, unless your veterinarian

instructs you otherwise. Typically, a multivitamin/ mineral supplement for cats contains all the B vitamins your cat needs. (See "Supplements for Your Cat" on p. 21.) The minimum requirement for kittens and cats for each of the B vitamins is as follows:

- **Thiamine (B_1):** 5.0 mg/kg
- **Riboflavin (B_2):** 4.0 mg/kg
- **Niacin (B_3):** 60.0 mg/kg
- **Pantothenic acid (B_5):** 5.0 mg/kg
- **B_6:** 4.0 mg/kg
- **Folic acid:** 0.8 mg/kg
- **Biotin:** 0.07 mg/kg
- **B_{12}:** 0.02 mg/kg

You may notice an unusually high amount of niacin in the above list. That's because cats are unable to synthesize a sufficient amount of niacin from the amino acid tryptophan the way many other mammals can. Therefore they need higher amounts in their diet. Cats who fail to get enough niacin can experience loss of appetite, weight loss, inflamed gums, and bloody diarrhea.

- **Vitamin D.** You can get your vitamin D from the sun when the ultraviolet rays convert vitamin D precursors in your skin into the active vitamin. Fluffy, however, isn't able to make this conversion efficiently, so she needs vitamin D in her diet. How does vitamin D help Fluffy? This nutrient plays a major role in regulating levels of calcium and phosphorus in the bloodstream, helps with bone formation, and is essential for nerve and muscle control. Kittens need 750 IU/kg, while grown cats require 500 IU/kg. If you give your cat a homemade diet, you may need to add vitamin D to the food, depending on the ingredients in the recipe.
- **Vitamin E.** This vitamin is also fat soluble, and it is found in high concentrations in liver, meats, and

fat, as well as in plant oils such as safflower and wheat germ. Cats need vitamin E to assist with fat metabolism, help form cell membranes, aid in cell respiration, and act as an antioxidant to prevent cell damage. Deficiencies of vitamin E are not uncommon in cats, especially those who are fed all-fish diets, which are naturally deficient in vitamin E. The daily minimum for kittens and cats is 30 IU/kg.

- **Vitamin K.** Cats are capable of making their own vitamin K. This vitamin is necessary for healthy blood function, including normal clotting. The main sources of vitamin K are egg yolk and green, leafy vegetables.

Minerals

The AAFCO has identified twelve minerals that are essential for cats: calcium, chloride, copper, iodine, iron, magnesium, manganese, phosphorus, potassium, selenium, sodium, and zinc. Your cat's diet should include all of these essential minerals, although it's not necessary that every meal meet these requirements. That said, you should strive to provide your kitty with all the essential minerals as often as possible, along with the other critical nutrients necessary for her health. If you give your cat a balanced diet using high-quality ingredients, you should have no problem providing the right amount of minerals. The value for each mineral provided here is the AAFCO minimum requirement and based on a dry-matter basis.

- **Calcium** is necessary for strong bones and teeth, blood coagulation, nerve impulse transmission, and healthy muscle contractions. The best food sources of calcium are bones, legumes, and dairy foods, while most meats and grains contain small amounts. Calcium works closely with phosphorus, and the correct calcium-to-phosphorus ratio is important for a cat's health. Cats needs slightly less phosphorus than they do calcium, so the ratio is around 1.2:1. Commercial cat food typically has calcium added, and if you make homemade food for your cat, you will need to add calcium as well. The AAFCO minimum is 1.0 mg/kg for kittens and 0.6 mg/kg for grown cats.

- **Chloride** is necessary for cats because it helps produce hydrochloric acid in the stomach, which aids in digestion, and also works with sodium to maintain the balance between the fluids inside and outside of cells. Mostly chloride works with sodium to form table salt. A chloride deficiency is extremely rare (see "Sodium" below). AAFCO minimum is 0.3 mg/kg.

- **Copper** is necessary for the formation of bone, collagen, and connective tissue, and it also helps the body absorb iron and develop red blood cells and the pigment in hair. Food sources of copper include liver, fish, whole grains, and legumes. The minimum daily requirement is 5.0 mg/kg, and the optimal form of copper is cuprous oxide or copper-lysine and not copper oxide if you are depending on supplementation in cat food products.

- **Iodine** is important for functioning of the thyroid gland and manufacture of thyroid hormones. This mineral is found mainly in fish and is added to commercial cat food in the form of potassium iodide potassium iodate, sodium iodide, or calcium iodate. The minimum requirement is 0.35 mg/kg based on dry matter.

- **Iron** is present in fish, lean meats, and liver, so an iron deficiency is uncommon unless you feed your cat a diet that does not provide an adequate amount of meat. Iron is necessary for the health and replenishment of red blood cells. The minimum amount of iron that cats need according to the AAFO is 80 mg/kg. Iron should be provided in forms other than iron oxide or iron carbonate.

- **Magnesium** plays many roles for your cat: It's necessary for the absorption and proper use of specific nutrients, such as vitamins C and E, and the minerals calcium, phosphorus, potassium, and sodium; it's required for proper bone growth; and it's needed for the functioning of enzymes. Magnesium is found in fish, milk, and whole grains, and the AAFCLO minimum requirement is 0.04 mg/kg.

- **Manganese** is involved in how the body uses carbohydrates and protein, reproduction, and the activity of enzymes that are responsible for the production of fatty acids and energy. Cats can get manganese from eggs, whole grains, and green vegetables, although many cat food makers add supplemental manganese to their products. Cats need a minimum of 7.5 mg/kg.

- **Phosphorus** works with calcium to support strong bones and teeth. It also has a role in energy metabolism, maintaining the acid-base balance, skeletal structure, and in DNA and RNA structure. Cats need 0.5 mg/kg while kittens require a minimum of 0.8 mg/kg.

- **Potassium** is required for the proper function of nerves, muscles, and enzymes, and to help keep the fluid in your cat's body in balance. Potassium is found in many foods so it's unusual for cats to experience a deficiency of this mineral. The AAFCO minimum requirement for potassium is 0.6 percent, although additional potassium may be needed if your cat is experiencing problems such as excessive diarrhea or vomiting, kidney disease, or other ailments that can cause a loss of potassium. Symptoms of potassium deficiency include nervous disorders, loss of appetite, poor growth, weakness, and cardiac arrest.

- **Selenium** is an antioxidant that works along with vitamin E to enhance the immune system and fight infections. Selenium is typically added to cat foods and is found in meat and cereals. The AAFCO minimum requirement is 0.1 mg/kg for both kittens and full-grown cats.

- **Sodium,** along with chloride, is necessary to help maintain proper fluid balance throughout the body, to transfer nutrients, and to remove waste products from cells. Generally, sodium and chloride not only work together, but they also are found together in many foods. The AAFO minimum requirement for sodium is 0.1 mg/kg. Generally, the requirement for chloride is 1.5 times that of sodium, because by weight salt provides 1.5 times more chloride than sodium.

- **Zinc** helps with protein metabolism and assists in wound healing, among other functions. The best food sources of zinc include red meat, whole grains, and peas. The AAFCO minimum requirement for zinc is 74.0 mg/kg on a dry-matter basis. Zinc deficiency in cats is not common, but kitties who have inflammatory bowel disease may experience zinc deficiency because they are not able to properly absorb the mineral.

SUPPLEMENTS FOR YOUR CAT

An estimated 33 percent of cats and dogs in the United States are given vitamins or other supplements, with multivitamins topping the list, followed by fatty acids and remedies for arthritis.

Why Cats Need Supplements

Basically, cats need supplements for the same reasons pet parents need them: to supplement a portion of their nutritional profile that is not being met by their diet and/or because they have a health condition that makes it necessary for them to take specific nutrients. Another category of cats who often need supplemenst are those who are pregnant or nursing, because they can develop nutritional deficiencies, especially if a cat becomes pregnant before she is a year old.

You will see many different supplements discussed in part II in individual chapters in the "Home Remedies" sections. Specific nutritional and herbal supplements can be helpful in managing a variety of symptoms and health problems.

Naturally, every cat has different needs, so not every cat should be given the same supplement, nor does every cat need the same supplement for any given condition or circumstance. If you choose to feed your cat homemade food, you will likely need to add supplements, even if you choose a raw-food diet. It is best to consult with your veterinarian or a feline nutritionist before giving supplements to your cat.

Finally, supplements—whether they are vitamins, minerals, herbs, enzymes, or other natural substances—can be helpful in managing a wide range of health challenges that your cat can face. You'll learn more about supplements used as home remedies in the chapters on cat conditions.

Do Supplements for Cats Work?

One question from pet parents regarding supplements is whether they really contain what is advertised on the label. The Food and Drug Administration oversees the quality of supplements for pets, but another organization—the National Animal Supplement Council—has the task of establishing labeling guidelines and testing supplements for pets to make sure they contain what they claim on the label. This nonprofit trade organization is made up of companies "committed to providing health supplements and nutritional supplements of the highest quality for companion animals, primarily dogs, cats and horses," according to their Web site.

Another question from pet parents is "Aren't nutritional supplements for my cat the same as the ones I'd take for myself?" The answer is no. (However, herbal remedies for people can be given to cats; see the introductory section to Part II.) Nutritional supplements for pets are typically formulated in ways that are specific for each animal, so it is best to choose supplements that have been formulated for cats if they are available. If nothing is on the market, then talk to your veterinarian about which human supplement is best.

How to Buy Cat Supplements

As your cat's health advocate and a supplement consumer, you should check on the quality of the ingredients in your cat's supplements. One unbiased resource to help you with that task is the ConsumerLab.com, an independent group that tests nutritional products and issues reports for the public. The ConsumerLab.com Web site allows you to access some information about supplements without charge, although there is a fee for some information (see the Appendix).

Here are some general guidelines for choosing quality supplements for your cat.

- ✓ **Look for products made by companies that have commissioned clinical studies of their supplements.**
- ✓ **Select a form your cat will take willingly—or at least with minimal resistance!** Cat supplements are often available in flavored chewable tablets, in liquid that can be added to food, or as a gel that can be placed on your cat's paw so she can lick it off.
- ✓ **Be familiar with the ingredients you want for your cat.** For example, there are several types of glucosamine: Which one is best for your cat?
- ✓ **If a supplement says it will prevent disease, be skeptical.** Such promises are too good to be true.
- ✓ **Select well-respected supplement makers.** These can include those offered by your veterinarian as well as others that have gotten good reports by ConsumerLab.com.
- ✓ **Look for products that provide a lot number (which indicates the company has quality control standards) and ways to contact the company.** Call

or send an e-mail to the company and ask about their product, such as if any studies have been done on the product and of you can see the study results for your review. Explore the manufacturer's Web site.
✓ **Look on the label for certification from an independent organization that has verified the contents of the supplement.**

Some cat food products, especially those formulated as therapeutic or prescription feline foods, contain specific supplements for particular conditions. For example, there are cat foods that contain glucosamine and chondroitin for kitties who are suffering with symptoms of osteoarthritis. Others may contain the omega-3 fatty acid DHA (docosahexaenoic acid) to help with cognitive dysfunction syndrome.

COMMON CAT SUPPLEMENTS

Here are some common nutritional supplements pet parents buy for their cats to supplement the food they provide. These supplements may be used as ingredients in homemade cat recipes or given as supplements at other times, such as after surgery or when recovering from an illness, either in food or alone. Several of these supplements also can be used to manage certain health conditions, and in those cases they are discussed in their appropriate individual chapters.

Multivitamins/Minerals

You may need to supplement your cat's food with a multivitamin/mineral supplement if you are making homemade cat food recipes and if your cat is eating commercial cat food. If you are feeding your cat a high-quality cat food that has extra vitamins and minerals or a food that has been prescribed by your veterinarian, talk to your vet before you give your cat any additional nutritional supplements, as they may not be necessary.

A good quality multivitamin/mineral should contain at least the essential vitamins, including vitamin A, D, E, and the B-complex vitamins (thiamine, riboflavin, niacin, B_5, B_6, folic acid, biotin, and B_{12}). Each of the individual ingredients in the multivitamin/mineral should come from natural, quality sources. If the sources are not revealed on the label, contact the company by phone or e-mail, or check their Web site to get the information. Examples of quality sources include cod liver oil, brewer's yeast, wheat germ, and liver.

Follow the dosing instructions on the supplement tube or bottle, which typically are given according to your cat's weight. For example, gels are often dosed by teaspoon or portions of a teaspoon, while chewable tablets are dosed by whole or half tablet per your cat's body weight.

Calcium

"Calcium is probably the most common deficiency in a homemade diet that isn't professionally balanced." That's the word from Claudia Kirk, DVM, PhD, a professor of medicine and nutrition at the University of Tennessee College of Veterinary Medicine. A professionally balanced homemade diet is one that has been developed or approved by a veterinarian or feline nutritionist.

Most, but not all, commercial cat foods provide a reasonable amount of calcium. If you give your cat homemade food that does not include ground bone, you will likely need to add a calcium supplement, which is easy to do (see "Make Your Own Calcium Supplement" below). Pregnant and nursing cats may need a calcium supplement as well.

You can make your own calcium supplement using eggshells. The best eggshells come from chickens that have been fed a natural (organic if possible) diet, because the shells reflect the nutrition provided to the birds. Eggshells contain calcium and about 25 other elements, such as boron, copper, iron, magnesium, manganese, molybdenum, silicon, sulfur, and zinc, among others.

MAKE YOUR OWN CALCIUM SUPPLEMENT

Save your egg shells and make your own calcium supplement for your cat. One eggshell from a medium egg provides about 1 teaspoon of powder. The calcium from egg shells balances the excess phosphorus in meat diets that do not include bone.

- Rinse eggshells in warm water and remove any egg white. Do not remove the papery membrane that is inside the eggshell, however, because it contains important nutrients.
- Dry the eggshells on a flat baking sheet, either in a low oven for 1 to 2 hours or in direct sunlight.
- Grind the eggshells in a clean blender, food processor, or coffee grinder.
- Sift through a very fine sieve and regrind any pieces left behind.
- Store the powdered eggshells in a container with a tight lid and keep it in a dry place.
- One-half teaspoon of finely ground eggshells provides approximately 1,000 mg of elemental calcium, or 400 mg of absorbable calcium.
- In a homemade diet recipe, you will need approximately ½ teaspoon of powdered eggshells for each pound of boneless meat.

Omega-3 Fatty Acid/Fish Oil Supplements

Omega-3 fatty acids are essential fatty acids, which means they must be obtained from the diet. These essential fatty acids play a significant role in protecting a cat's immune system, eyes, brain, liver, and joints. Although commercial cat food often contains some omega-3s, some pet parents and veterinarians believe their cats do not get enough omega-3s from these foods.

In fact, there are no official recommendations for the amount of omega-3 fatty acids a cat's diet should contain, and cat food makers are not required to list the amount of omega-3 contained in their products. If this sounds like a guessing game, you're right! If you feed your cat a homemade diet, then you may need to supplement with a fish oil supplement (omega-3 fatty acids are mainly found in fish oil), depending on the ingredients you choose for your cat's diet.

The two main omega-3 fatty acids are EPA (eicosapentaenoic acid) and DHA (docosahexaenoic acid), and both are found in cold water fish such as tuna, herring, salmon, and mackerel—foods cats love! EPA and DHA work together to reduce inflammation and support other health-related benefits.

If you choose an omega-3 fatty acid supplement for your cat, look for regular fish oil or salmon oil. Avoid cod liver oil supplements because they are typically high in vitamins A and D, which often are not necessary to provide as a supplement and can be toxic at high amounts. Some cod liver oil supplements advertise themselves as being low in vitamins A and D; however, these should be used with caution.

Some pet parents ask whether they can give their cat omega-3 fatty acids in the form of flaxseed oil. The omega-3 in flaxseed oil is called alpha-linolenic acid (ALA), and cats have very limited ability to convert ALA to EPA, which must be done before the body can use the omega-3s. Therefore, it's best to supplement with fish or salmon oil rather than flaxseed oil.

The suggested dose of fish oil for cats is about 750 mg (from a supplement that contains a combination of EPA and DHA) per 10 pounds of body weight. However, the dose depends on whether you are supplementing the diet or giving the fish oil to help manage symptoms or a health problem. In the latter case, the dose is typically higher. Amounts of omega-3 fatty acids given for specific health conditions differ from these maintenance levels and are explained in their appropriate chapters.

Fish oil is available as a liquid and in gel capsules. The gel caps are easy to pierce with a needle, which allows you to squeeze out the oil into your cat's food.

HOW MUCH FOOD DOES MY CAT NEED?

How much food should you feed your cat? In reality, no one really knows. Every cat is different, and unfortunately you can't count on the instructions on the cans and bags of cat food you buy at the store to accurately guide you. How much food you feed your cat depends on your cat's health, her age, her breed, her level of activity, what type of food you are feeding her, whether your cat is overweight and needs to lose weight, and how well you are meeting her nutritional needs. So although I'd love to tell you exactly how much you should feed your cat, I can't.

That said, what I can tell you is that it's a matter of trial and error. Take an honest look at your cat's weight and what he or she should weigh. In chapter 16 you can learn more about obesity in cats and how to solve the problem, but for now, here's how to determine how much to feed your cat.

First, consider how much your cat *should* weigh. Although you may think Ginger looks healthy with a round, Garfield-like face and chubby belly, she is likely overweight, and what you feed her is probably keeping her that way. Generally, a mixed breed domestic cat should weigh between 8 and 11 pounds (with females at the lower end of the range), while Siamese should weigh between 5 and 10 pounds, Persians should weigh about 10 pounds, and Maine coons should weigh between 11 and 15 pounds, according to the Association for Pet Obesity Prevention (APOP).

If you think you can depend on what the commercial cat food labels say about feeding your cat, don't. Their recommendations are questionable at best, and are designed to lull you into buying more cat food. Cat food makers may overstate or understate how much food to feed cats, depending on whether they want to sell more cat food or try to make their product look like it's a better deal than their competitors'. They also do not know your cat.

So how much food should you feed your cat? The average 10-pound cat should eat between 180 and 200 calories per day and get about thirty minutes of exercise daily to maintain weight, according to the APOP. If Ginger weighs 15 pounds, she needs to lose a few pounds. The amount of food Ginger needs is probably around 225 to 250 calories per day if you want to reduce her weight to 12 pounds. Unless you know how many calories are in the amount of food you are now feeding Ginger, you will need to experiment with the amount of food you are feeding her, weigh her every week (a digital scale is best), and gradually make adjustments to the amount of food you feed. Yes, it takes time and effort, but the reward is a healthier cat and a good chance of lower vet bills.

To help you calculate the number of calories in any specific wet or dry cat food, there is a calculator available online: http://www.knowyourcat.info/calorycalc.htm. The calculator allows you to enter the amount of protein, fat, ash, moisture, and fiber as stated on the cat food label, and the calculator will then determine for you the number of calories per 100 grams of food. Although cat food labels don't reveal the amount of carbohydrates in the food (which is important information for pet parents to have), the calculator also provides that information as well.

For example, I compared two different brands of canned cat food (one a well-known brand available in most grocery stores and the other a generic brand) and one well-known, higher-end brand of dry cat food available in grocery stores. Here's the comparison.

- **Well-known canned brand.** First three ingredients are tuna, water, and egg bits: a minimum of 14 percent protein, a minimum 2 percent fat, a maximum 1 percent fiber, a maximum 3 percent ash, and a maximum 78 percent moisture. The calculation reveals that the canned food contains 73 calories per 100 grams of food. Since the canned food contains 156 grams (5.5 oz), the entire can holds approximately 110 calories. It also reveals that the food provides 67.1 percent of calories from protein, 23.2 percent from fat, and 9.58 percent from carbohydrates. All three factors are within the healthy range for cats.

- **Generic canned brand.** First three ingredients are ocean fish, water, and poultry by-products. Minimum protein is 11 percent, minimum fat 3 percent, maximum fiber 1.5 percent, maximum ash 3.5 percent, and maximum moisture 78 percent. The calculation reveals that this food provides 49.3 percent of calories from protein, 32.6 percent from fat, and 17.9 percent from carbohydrates. The 78 calories per 100 grams translates into about 120 calories per 5.5-ounce can. The carbohydrates in this canned food are higher than desirable and the protein content is marginal. However, as you will notice, even this generic canned food provides better nutrition than the well-known dry-cat-food brand (below).

- **Well-known dry brand.** The first three ingredients were salmon, brewer's rice, and corn gluten meal: a minimum of 34 percent protein, a minimum of 13 percent fat, a maximum of 2.5 percent fiber, and a maximum of 12 percent moisture. The calculation revealed that 100 grams of this food provided 366 calories, with carbohydrates making up 37.2 percent of the calories—way above the 5 percent recommended for cats. Protein made up 32.5 percent of calories, while fat made up 30.1 percent. Because of the high carbohydrate content, this dry food not only provides too many calories, it also does not give your cat enough protein or fat.

The bottom line when it comes to how much to feed your cat is this: Know how much your cat should weigh, determine how much food she needs to eat at her ideal weight, and choose nutritious foods to meet those needs.

In this chapter I emphasized the importance of choosing wet food over dry, but there is another choice, and that's homemade cat food, which allows you to control the quality and quantity of ingredients. Homemade cat food is discussed throughout the rest of this book, including tips and recipes on how to prepare quick, quality food for your cat.

First, however, you should learn more about commercial cat foods and why they often are not the best way to feed your cat.

Chapter 2

Cat Food: You Expect Me to Eat This?

If cats could talk—and many pet parents will argue that they can—they would probably tell you what they think about the commercial cat food you may be feeding them. The food you choose to give to your cat has a tremendous impact on her overall health and whether she will develop a wide spectrum of symptoms, ailments, and diseases. The equations are simple: poor quality food = significant risk of poor health; high-quality food = significant chance of a healthy, happy cat.

This chapter looks at commercial cat food and helps you sift through what's on the shelf. It also answers the following questions: Who sets cat food standards? What is in commercial cat food? Which types of commercial cat foods are good for your cat? How can you decipher cat food labels?

THE BUSINESS OF FEEDING KITTY

The pet food industry is big business, and it's a business that doesn't necessarily have the health and well-being of your cat at heart. In fact, most commercial pet food makers use "feed grade" ingredients that don't meet the same standards as the food you eat. One striking example is the source of animal protein in pet food, and since cats get—or should get—the majority of their calories from animal protein, this is an area of concern for pet parents.

Some of the ingredients used within the pet food industry comes from "4-D" livestock—dead, diseased, dying, and disabled. There are even reports—denied by the industry, of course—of the use of euthanized dogs and cats as well as roadkill and zoo animals. The motive is simple: These ingredients are cheap and they are technically sources of protein, as distressing as this fact may be. These animals also may be rendered into liquid or dry by-products and added to "enhance" the palatability of the food.

Other cat food ingredients are also often of low or questionable quality. Cheap fillers such as ground corn, corn gluten, soybean and peanut hulls, and wheat and soybean flours—all of which are often seen in dry cat foods, the vast majority of which should not be fed to cats—are common ingredients as well. The icing on the cake, so to speak, are the additives: artificial colors and flavors, preservatives, antibiotics, and hormones that are not meant for feline consumption. The end result is food not fit for your cat.

There is good news, however, and it comes from two sources. One is that there are some cat food producers who make whole, natural, and even organic high-quality products for cats. These products typically are not available in standard grocery stores but can be found in pet stores, on the Internet, and from some veterinarians. (See "High-Quality Commercial Cat Food" on page 41.) Another source is homemade cat food, which is covered in chapter 3, "What's for Dinner? Good Food for Your Cat."

CAT FOOD STANDARDS: AAFCO

The Association of American Feed Control Officials (AAFCO) establishes the nutritional standards that it has deemed to be complete and balanced for pet foods. In each state, it is the feed control official's responsibility to make sure the laws established to protect pet food are followed, and those regulations say only unadulterated food that has been properly and uniformly labeled should be made available to the marketplace. However, it is the responsibility of the pet food companies to make their products according to the AAFCO standards. The AAFCO does not test, regulate, approve, or certify pet foods in any way.

The following is a portion of the AAFCO nutritional standards for kittens and cats as established the by AAFCO's Feline Nutrition Expert Subcommittee. The levels of nutrients in the chart are expressed on a "dry-matter" basis. However, when you read a cat food label, the amounts stated on the "Guaranteed Analysis" section of the product are given on an "as fed" basis. This means you need to pull out your pocket calculator and convert "as fed" to "dry matter." Here's how to do it.

Let's start with dry cat food. If the label says it contains 10 percent moisture, that means it has 90 percent dry matter. Now choose a nutrient; let's say protein. If the label says the food contains 22 percent protein, divide the 22 percent protein by the 90 percent dry matter, and you get 24 percent. This is the amount of protein in the food on a dry-matter basis. You can now compare the dry food with a canned food. The label reads "max. 78%," which means the maximum dry matter is 22 percent. The label also says "crude protein minimum 9%." Take the 9 percent and divide it by 22 percent to get the percentage of protein on a dry-matter basis, which in this case is about 40 percent.

You can use the same formula to figure out how much fat and fiber are in the cat foods you are considering.

Where Are the Carbs?

You may have noticed in the above explanation about cat food that there was no mention of carbohydrates. Pet food makers do not provide information on carbohydrate content, however, and that's too bad for pet parents and convenient for pet food manufacturers. Why?

Because most commercial cat foods—primarily dry foods but also some brands of canned foods—provide excessive amounts of carbohydrates. If you read the section about carbohydrates in chapter 1, you already know that carbohydrates are not only unnatural for cats but also pose significant health risks. Yet carbohydrates—corn and cornmeal, soybean meal, wheat, hulls, and more—are cheap ingredients and cheap fillers. Combine these facts with the convenience offered by providing your cat dry cat food—just put it in the bowl and forget it—and you have the ingredients for a product that cat food makers can easily market to pet parents and make a profit, but at the expense of your cat's health.

AAFCO NUTRITIONAL STANDARDS FOR KITTENS AND CATS

Note: This represents a selected number of nutrients from the AAFCO list; it is not the entire table. All figures are given on a dry matter basis.

Nutrient	Kitten	Cat
Protein	30%	26%
Fat	9%	9%
Calcium	1.0%	0.6%
Phosphorus	0.8%	0.5%
Potassium	0.6%	0.6%
Sodium	0.2%	0.2%
Chloride	0.3%	0.3%
Magnesium	0.08%	0.04%
Iron	80.0 mg/kg	80.0 mg/kg
Copper	5.0 mg/kg	5.0 mg/kg
Manganese	7.5 mg/kg	7.5 mg/kg
Iodine	0.35 mg/kg	0.35 mg/kg
Selenium	0.1 mg/kg	0.1 mg/kg
Zinc	75.0 mg/kg	75.0 mg/kg

HOW TO READ CAT FOOD LABELS

As you discovered in chapter 1 under "How Much Food Does My Cat Need?" cat food labels provide cryptic nutritional information on the minimum levels of crude protein and crude fat, and the maximum levels of crude fiber and moisture. They also may list maximum ash, minimum taurine, and other nutrients. This nutritional information is provided under the heading "Guaranteed Analysis," which food manufacturers are legally required to provide.

But what about the ingredients in cat food? If a canned food provides your cat with 55 percent of calories as protein, what are the sources of that protein? The same goes for the fat and the "hidden" carbohydrates.

When you look at the ingredient panel on human food, the order the ingredients are listed on the label is by weight, and the same is true for cat food. For example, if the first ingredient on the cat food label is chicken, you can assume the product is providing a high-quality source of protein. However, if the first ingredient is meat meal, the protein quality is much less. If the first ingredient is corn gluten, put that product back on the shelf, because what you have in your hands is a high-carbohydrate food not suitable for your kitty.

However, cat food makers can be a bit devious. Let's say the first ingredient is turkey. Good so far. But if the next two or three ingredients are some variation of a carbohydrate, such as corn gluten, cornmeal, and ground yellow corn, the combination of those three corn sources is greater than the first listed ingredient. Therefore, while at first it appears you have a cat food whose main ingredient is turkey, you really have a product that is mostly corn. It pays to read labels carefully and read between the lines, so to speak.

CAT FOOD INGREDIENTS

Here is another dilemma you face when looking at cat food labels: the exact identity of the ingredients. Do you know what chicken by-products are? How about meat meal? And why does cat food need to contain soybean hulls? In addition to ingredients with words that sound like food, there are also those representing artificial ingredients, preservatives, and chemicals. Most cat foods contain these nonfood items, and all of them must be approved by the FDA or be designated "generally recognized as safe" (GRAS). In addition, cat food producers are required to list the preservatives on the label, even though they do not always list those that have been processed somewhere else (e.g., China) and then added to their products.

Your cat doesn't need artificial colors, flavors, preservatives, and other chemicals in her food, so if you choose commercial cat foods, look for those that are all natural. (See "High-Quality Commercial Cat Food" on page 41 for suggestions.) When it comes to added nutrients, select products that use natural nutrients, such as ascorbic acid for vitamin C and mixed tocopherols for vitamin E. Because cat foods made with natural ingredients and without preservatives have a shorter shelf life than foods made with chemicals, check the product for an expiration date.

Here is a list of some of the ingredients you can find in most commercial cat foods. These descriptions are based mainly on information from the AAFCO.

- **Animal digest.** This is the liquid that results when clean animal tissue is cooked down. Animal digest is not supposed to come from the use of hair, teeth, hooves, feathers, or horns except in trace amounts that might unavoidably be added during processing.
- **Animal fat.** A byproduct of the tissues of animals obtained during meat processing.

- **Artificial colors and flavors.** These might be better called "mystery ingredients." Cat food makers are allowed to state "added color" or "artificial and natural flavors" on the label without naming the sources. These additives provide no nutritional value and may be harmful to your cat's health.
- **Ascorbic acid.** This is another name for vitamin C and can help with metabolism.
- **Beet pulp.** This dried residue from sugar beets provides fiber but is also high in sugar and should be avoided.
- **BHA/BHT.** Butylated hydroxyanisole (BHA) and butylated hydroxytoluene (BHT) are preservatives typically used in dry cat food to protect fats from turning rancid. Many countries have banned BHA and BHT, but not the United States. Research shows that high levels of BHA and BHT can promote or contribute to cancer, kidney and liver damage, dry skin, and dental disease in animals.
- **Corn bran.** Corn bran is the outer coating of the corn kernel and provides carbohydrates. It is a common filler that has minimal nutritional value.
- **Corn gluten meal.** After removing most of the starch and germ from corn, what remains can be dried and made into corn gluten meal, which is a low-quality protein source and a carbohydrate your cat does not need.
- **Corn syrup.** The concentrated juice extracted from corn.
- **Dried whey.** The substance that remains after removing water from whey, which is the watery part of milk. Dried whey contains not less than 11 percent protein nor less than 61 percent lactose.
- **Ethoxyquin.** A preservative that prevents fats from turning rancid. The FDA asked pet food manufacturers to reduce by 50 percent the maximum levels of ethoxyquin allowed in food after research showed the preservative might cause liver damage in animals

who consumed high levels. Ethoxyquin is also associated with reproductive problems, cancer, organ failure, and skin allergies.

- **Fish meal.** Clean, dried, and ground tissue of undecomposed whole fish or fish pieces. The fish oil may or may not have been removed. Fish meal is considered to be an excellent source of omega-3 fatty acids.

- **Gelatin.** A colorless, nearly tasteless and odorless substance that is made by boiling bones, animal skin, and connective tissue. Gelatin is a binding agent used in cat food and also a source of protein.

- **Ground yellow corn.** A common ingredient in dry cat food and an inexpensive filler. Corn also is a common allergen and can be difficult for cats to digest.

- **Linoleic acid.** An essential fatty acid (omega-6) found in most vegetable oils. Linoleic acid may appear on the label as soybean oil, lecithin, corn oil, linseed oil, or wheat germ oil.

- **Meat.** Meat is the clean flesh of slaughtered animals and can include skeletal muscle, diaphragm, heart, esophagus, tongue, overlying fat, and part of the skin, nerves, sinew, and blood vessels normally in the flesh. However, the FDA does not allow pet food to contain body parts from animals who have tested positive for mad cow disease, nor can it include brains or spinal cords from older animals, who are at higher risk of the disease.

- **Meat by-products.** According to the AAFCO, meat by-products can include the blood, liver, brains, bone, udders, lungs, ligaments, stomach, and intestines. It is not supposed to contain beaks, hair, teeth, horns, or hooves, although some reports claim that it does.

- **Meat meal.** Rendered meal made from animal tissue. It is not supposed to contain blood, hair, hooves, horns, hide trimmings, stomach contents, or manure, although any of these substances that get into the meal unavoidably during processing are allowed.

- **Natural flavors.** Flavor ingredients that are minimally processed and do not contain artificial or synthetic components.
- **Poultry by-products.** Clean parts of slaughtered poultry, including the heart, lungs, liver, kidneys, feet, abdomen, heads, and intestines (free of feces or foreign matter).
- **Poultry by-product meal.** This ingredient consists of the ground, rendered, and clean parts of slaughtered poultry, including the feet, neck, intestines, and undeveloped eggs. Feathers are not allowed except for those that may unavoidably enter during processing.
- **Rice gluten meal.** The dried remains after most of the starch and germ are removed from rice. Rice gluten meal is a carbohydrate cats do not need.
- **Soybean hulls.** The outer covering of soybeans, it is a source of fiber but also used as a cheap filler.
- **Soybean meal (de-hulled, solvent extracted).** Meal obtained by grinding the soybean flakes that remain after most of the oil has been removed from de-hulled soybeans using a solvent extraction process.

SECRET CODE WORDS ON CAT FOOD LABELS

Did you know that:

- When cat food makers use the word "with" on the label—as in "Rice with Beef"—it means that the product is required to contain only 3 percent of the "with" ingredient. Therefore "Rice with Beef" is mainly rice.
- Cat foods that use the word "flavor" are not required to have any of the ingredient in the product. So if the label says "beef flavor," the cat

food manufacturer is not required to include any beef in the product.

- Words like "recipe," "formula," and "dinner" are a sneaky way of saying that the ingredient named in the cat food makes up one-quarter of the food. For example, if you buy "Chicken Dinner for Kitty," only 25 percent of the total ingredients is chicken. Be sure to read the ingredient label carefully.

HIGH-QUALITY COMMERCIAL CAT FOOD

Identifying high-quality commercial cat foods is not an easy task, because you must put aside the marketing hype and try to decipher what is *really* in the products. I depended on several sources for my search, including input from various experts and Web sites, including but not limited to Lisa Pierson, DVM; Susan Thixton (Truth About Pet Food); Petfoodtalk.com; Consumersearch.com; and the individual Web sites for dozens of cat food makers, the vast majority of whom offer ingredient and Guaranteed Analysis information for each product on their pages. This allowed me to analyze individual products for protein, fat, and carbohydrate content. I focused on canned food but did calculate protein/fat/carbohydrate content for a few dry food items as well.

I found that even among high-priced items boasting all-natural ingredients with no fillers, preservatives, by-products, antibiotics, and/or hormones, frequently there were cat foods that were too high in carbohydrate content (25 percent or higher) and, correspondingly, too low in protein. Some were excessively high in fat. However, this was not always true for every item offered by a manufacturer. That means you need to check each item if you want to find the ones that provide the high-protein/low-carbohydrate balance that is best for your cat.

The bottom line is, the following alphabetical list of cat

food makers represents those that *generally* offer high-quality cat food. All of them use human-grade meats, fowl, and fish, and their other ingredients are also high-quality. Two of the entries offer organic foods, and they are marked as such, and one entry provides a raw food diet. Most offer grain-free products, but remember that a small amount of high-quality grain is okay. I have indicated the one cat food producer who appears to be the best of the bunch; however, this is not in any way an endorsement. The best food in the world for cats is useless unless Mr. Whiskers (or whoever your cat is) agrees to eat it.

- **Blue Buffalo and Blue Organic.** Two brand lines by the same manufacturer, with organic offerings.
- **Feline's Pride.** This is a raw cat food containing less than 1 percent carbohydrates and fortified with taurine and other nutrients.
- **Freshpet.** Offers a refrigerated line of fresh cat food.
- **Merrick Pet Care.** Offers grain-free products.
- **Natura Pet.** Offers grain-free varieties.
- **Natural Balance.** Offers some limited ingredient products for cats with special needs, in addition to a regular product line.
- **Newman's Own Organics.** The name says it all. The foods do contain some grains.
- **Wellness.** Most of their offerings are grain-free.
- **Weruva.** Grain-free. Superior when it comes to high levels of protein and very low carbohydrates.

Chapter 3
What's for Dinner? Good Food for Your Cat

Now that you've read about the types of nutrients your cat needs for optimal health and the products offered by the commercial cat food manufacturers, it's time to add yet another element to the dietary picture: homemade food for your cat. This chapter offers suggestions on how you can provide your kitty with convenient, nutritious, cost-effective food that will support and maintain her health. Here you will learn which specific foods are good for your cat, the benefits they provide, and how you can use them to prepare simple homemade meals your cat will love. Whether you make the switch to homemade meals for your cat all the time or several times a week—or use homemade recipes occasionally to mix with high-quality wet cat foods on the market—this chapter will help you answer your cat when she looks at you with that question in her eyes: *What's for dinner?*

WHY HOMEMADE FOOD?

Which would you rather have, a bowl of dried, processed cereal or a stack of homemade whole-grain pancakes with fresh fruit? A dish of processed pasta from a can or a home-cooked plate of penne with fresh marinara sauce? You already know that fresh, whole foods are best for your health, and the same is true for your cat. So why place a bowl of chemically laden dried food in front of her every day?

Homemade food is a healthful alternative to the vast field of poor-quality commercial cat foods on the market. While many commercial foods can cause allergic reactions and contribute to the development of health problems such as dermatitis, kidney failure, obesity, and diabetes, offering your cat homemade foods gives you control over the quality and nutritional value of your cat's diet and how the food is prepared. You can eliminate the additives and chemicals that pose health risks to your cat and make modifications to each recipe to fit his needs, depending on his weight, health problems, allergies, and amount of exercise.

Understand that just because something is homemade doesn't mean it's nutritious. You must use fresh, wholesome ingredients, and cats especially need high-quality protein. However, with a minimum amount of effort, you can create homemade food your cat can enjoy at every meal or to complement high-quality commercial food, and it need not cost you any more than high-quality commercial food—and will likely cost you less. One simple secret is to prepare a large batch of any given recipe each time and freeze individual portions. Then you'll have plenty of food on hand that may last for days, weeks, even several months. What will last even longer, however, is the satisfaction of knowing you are providing sound nutrition for your cat.

RAW DIET VERSUS COOKED

One topic of debate and disagreement among veterinarians is the raw food diet. Some experts, like Cathy Alinovi, DVM, a practicing veterinarian, certified veterinarian food therapist, and author of *Dinner PAWsible: A Cookbook for Healthy Dog & Cat Meals*, believe raw makes sense (although the recipes in her book are cooked). "For an adult cat's diet, raw meat is close to all that's needed," she is quoted in a Consumer Media Network article. She and other raw diet advocates point out that cats are natural carnivores and that a raw-food diet, when made with high-quality ingredients and handled properly, is the most beneficial diet for kitties.

Others voice concerns about contamination from bacteria, parasites, and other factors. And there are certainly those pet parents who do not want to handle a raw food diet for personal or ethical reasons.

So far, few scientific studies have adequately explored the topic of raw food diets for cats. In one of the few published studies, which appeared in the January 2011 issue of the *Canadian Veterinary Journal*, the authors concluded that "there is some compelling evidence suggesting that raw food diets may be a theoretical risk nutritionally" and that "raw food poses a substantial risk of infectious disease to the pet, the pet's environment, and the humans in the household." At the same time, they did not turn their backs on a raw-food diet completely. "Although there is a lack of large cohort studies to evaluate risk or benefit of raw meat diets fed to pets," they continued, "there is enough evidence to compel veterinarians to discuss human health implications of these diets with owners."

In a subsequent study done at the University of Illinois, the investigators compared raw diets and cooked diets for cats and evaluated their nutritional value and digestibility. They concluded, in their own words, that "cooking a raw meat diet does not alter apparent total tract energy and macronutrient digestibility and may also minimize risk of microbial contamination." They also pointed out that, since there is a growing interest in raw-food diets for cats, "further research focused on the adequacy and safety of raw beef-based diets in domestic cats is justified."

If a raw-food diet is something you want to consider, organic meats are recommended to help prevent potential problems associated with consuming raw foods. Here are some factors you should consider.

- **Cost.** Organic meats are expensive and not always readily available.
- **Handling.** Some pet parents are not comfortable handling raw meat, whether it's the ick factor, ethical reasons, or something else.
- **Digestion.** Although cats in the wild naturally eat raw meat, some of today's domesticated felines have

difficulty digesting raw meats and experience gastrointestinal problems such as vomiting, diarrhea,
and loose stools when on a raw diet.

- **Parasites.** Raw meat can contain the eggs and larvae of parasites, which can be destroyed when foods
are cooked properly. Freezing some meats may destroy some but not all parasites.

- **Bacteria.** Bacterial contamination of meat, fowl,
and even produce is often in the news, and the risk
of harmful exposure to these microorganisms,
such as salmonella and E. coli, is greatest in raw
foods.

- **Human contamination.** Cats who consume bacteria can pass the organisms into the environment,
where they can infect you and your family. You also
may contaminate your own food if you handle raw
meats and do not properly wash your hands, food
preparation surfaces, utensils, and dishes.

Before making a switch to a raw food diet for your cat,
consider the risks and benefits and consult several experts.
Even if you decide to "go raw" as a special treat for your cat,
it still pays to know the hazards.

A GROCERY LIST FOR YOUR CAT

It's time to make a grocery list for your cat and pick out the
foods that are both good for him and that you can use to prepare some simple meals. Your kitty shopping list may look
surprisingly like the one for you and your family (depending
on your eating habits; my apologies to vegetarians), and after
all, your cat *is* a member of your family.

The following list of foods are those that are safe and
nutritious for cats. Since kitties are finicky creatures, chances
are your cat will not like everything on this list, and in some
cases, depending on health issues, not every food will be

suitable. However, with such a wide selection, there's sure to be plenty your cat will enjoy.

Animal Protein

Beef

Beef is a high-protein source that provides B vitamins, iron, selenium, phosphorus, and zinc. Ground beef comes in a form that frees you from grinding it. Most supermarkets sell three or four grades of ground beef based on the amount of fat they contain, ranging from 93 percent lean/7 percent fat to about 73 percent lean/27 percent fat. Because cats need a fair amount of fat, the 7 percent fat is too lean unless you are adding some fat to the recipe. If you buy beef in forms other than ground, cut off excess fat and grind the meat in a meat grinder or food processor.

Chicken

Chicken is both a good source of protein and a fairly inexpensive form of protein. Ground chicken, which is about 15 percent fat, is usually priced higher. Organic chicken is best, but it is more expensive. Skinless chicken breast contains only about 1 percent fat, while thigh meat has a higher fat content and is therefore better for cats. However, some cats prefer white meat, while others like the darker flesh, so you may need to experiment. If your cat likes only the breast, add the skin when you grind it to add some fat. You may also want to add finely ground raw chicken bones to the ground chicken. Be sure the bones are finely ground before you mix them with the ground chicken and feed it to your cat.

Turkey

Turkey pieces and ground turkey are typically well liked by cats. The darker meat has more fat and so is a better choice. Ground turkey is usually sold in three grades: 1, 7, and 15 percent fat. If you decide to grind turkey bones, be sure you have a good grinder, as they can be tough to process.

Fish and Seafood

It's hard to find a cat who doesn't like some kind of fish or seafood. Look for wild-caught cold-water fish, such as salmon, sardines, halibut, orange roughy, tuna, and mackerel. Of pond-raised fish, U.S.-produced catfish may be safe and reasonably priced. These fish are all excellent sources of protein and omega-3 fatty acids, which help the skin, fur, and immune system. Although no fish are free of some type of contaminant, farm-raised fish are typically a poor choice because they have been fed antibiotics to help prevent disease. Organically raised fish are in limited supply.

Feel free to finely grind up the bones and add them to the cooked fish when feeding your cat, as the bones are an excellent source of calcium. Cooked rather than raw fish is recommended. In the seafood department, cats enjoy shrimp and clams.

A few cautionary words about feeding your cat fish. Because fish often harbor mercury and other toxic chemicals and heavy metals, limit the amount of fish you feed your kitty to about two days per week. Also, avoid giving your cat canned tuna designed for people, except as an occasional treat. Too much canned tuna, especially if it is the main food, can harm your cat because (1) tuna, especially albacore, often contains mercury; (2) tuna doesn't contain taurine, which cats require; and (3) tuna also is short on copper, iron, calcium, and vitamins A, B, and E.

Organ Meats

Chicken liver is a very rich source of vitamin A and an excellent way to provide your kitty with B vitamins (e.g., thiamine, riboflavin, niacin, pantothenic acid, and folic acid), and vitamin K, as well as iron. However, chicken liver should be doled out in small amounts because too much vitamin A can be toxic in cats, who store the fat-soluble vitamin in their liver. For example, one of the recipes at the end of this chapter contains 2 tablespoons of cooked, ground chicken liver, which is the total amount for one 10-pound cat for one day. Chicken kidney and heart should be fed in a similar way.

Dairy Case

Eggs

Eggs are the most easily digested form of protein for your cat, as well as the highest quality of protein. In fact, eggs are the gold standard for protein, with a 100 rating, while meats, fish, and fowl are all lower in quality (see chapter 1 for the discussion on protein). When giving eggs to your cat, make sure they are cooked. Share some of your scrambled eggs with your kitty! Avoid raw eggs, as raw egg whites contain an enzyme called avidin, which reduces the absorption of the B vitamin biotin. A deficiency of biotin can cause skin and haircoat problems. Cooked egg whites can be a critical part of the diet of a cat who has chronic kidney failure (see chapter 15). In addition to protein, eggs are a great source of ribo-flavin, selenium, and the fat-soluble vitamins A, D, E, and K.

Milk and Cheese

Dairy foods like milk and cheese are a good source of protein and calcium, but those made from cows' milk also contain lactose, a sugar that some cats cannot tolerate or digest well. If your cat can tolerate dairy products (she will experience di-arrhea and/or gas within 8 to 12 hours if she cannot), there's really no need to feed her these foods too often or in more than tiny amounts. Two dairy products that are low in lactose are farmer cheese and dry cottage cheese, which you can offer as a treat on occasion. An alternative is to freeze cottage cheese and pour off the liquid that gathers on top as it thaws. The liquid contains most of the lactose. As for kittens, do not give them cow's milk. Even though kittens do have the enzyme (lactase) necessary to deal with lactose, they don't have enough to handle the high levels of lactose found in cow's milk.

Yogurt

Small amounts of plain yogurt are okay for your cat if she is not lactose intolerant, but do not choose brands that contain sugars, artificial sweeteners, or any type of fat substitutes (e.g., Simplesse, Olestra). The best thing about yogurt is the live bacteria, as these beneficial organisms can help keep your cat's intestinal tract in balance and support the immune system. Yogurt is also a good source of calcium.

Grains, Legumes, and Seeds

Cats do not need much in the way of carbohydrates, but limited amounts of certain foods can add essential nutrients and variety to their diet. Among the carbohydrates cats can enjoy are certain grains, legumes, and seeds.

- Ground flax seed is a rich source of omega-3 fatty acids, which benefit your cat's skin and haircoat, help with allergy symptoms, and provide a source of fiber. You can grind raw flax seed in a coffee grinder or food processor to add to your cat's food and store the remainder in a tightly sealed dark container in the refrigerator.
- Legumes, including beans, lentils, and split peas, are a source of both protein and fiber, along with iron, phosphorus, folate, thiamine, magnesium, manganese, and molybdenum, which has a role in detoxifying the body.
- Brown rice is an ingredient you often see in cat food, and you can add it to your recipes as well, although not in the amounts typically seen in commercial cat foods. Brown rice provides a fair amount of fiber, protein, iron, calcium, and phosphorus. Skip the white stuff and go brown.
- Oatmeal in tiny amounts is okay to add, especially if your kitty needs a little fiber boost because of hairballs or constipation. If you do give your cat oatmeal, be sure it's cooked and made without sugar or other additives.
- Amaranth and quinoa, two grain-like foods that are high in protein and gluten-free, also are healthful additions in small amounts.

• Wheat can be an allergen, but some cats do fine with a small amount of pasta as part of their meal.

Vegetables and Fruits

A small amount of vegetables and fruit are healthful for cats, but just don't overdo it. That means perhaps a tablespoon or two maximum per day for variety. The vegetables can be cooked or raw, depending on how they are usually served, and should be either finely chopped or mashed. Veggies are generally a good source of vitamins, minerals, and phytonutrients, along with fiber. Check out the recipes in this chapter and elsewhere for vegetable ideas. Cats are less likely to eat fruit, especially since they do not have taste receptors for sweet.

Vegetables you can add to your cat's food—and that they might eat—include bell peppers, carrots, broccoli, cauliflower, green beans, summer and winter squash, pumpkin, sweet peas, sweet potatoes, and white potatoes.

SIMPLE RULES OF HOMEMADE CAT FOOD

When you prepare homemade cat food, there are three simple but critical rules to remember, according to Cathy Alinovi, DVM, certified in veterinary food therapy and author of *Dinner PAWSible: A Cookbook for Healthy Dog & Cat Meals*: Use quality ingredients, strive for overall balance, and make a variety of recipes. I will also mention a few of the "minor" rules concerning doubling and tripling recipes, storage, and serving suggestions. Let's start with the main rules.

Quality Ingredients

One of the main reasons to make homemade cat food is to control the quality, so you need to start with high-quality ingredients. This rule applies especially to your protein sources, as they make up the majority of the meal. You know what quality ingredients are: natural, whole foods, organic if possible. You want to avoid refined, processed foods, including those that contain artificial ingredients and preservatives, sugars, and high sodium. Refer to the list of different foods you can use in your recipes, the recipes in this chapter and in others throughout the book, and those you get from your veterinarian or feline nutritionist. (For a list of specific foods to avoid, see the Appendix.)

Overall Balance

The overall balance rule works in tandem with the next rule: variety. First of all, cats need lots of protein (at least 50 to 60 percent), a moderate amount of fat (about 30 percent), and a small amount of carbohydrates (5 to 10 percent is best). They also need a variety of vitamins, minerals, and other nutrients as already discussed in chapter 1. However, every meal you feed your cat will probably not meet every single macronutrient and micronutrient need for your cat.

Are every one of your meals nutritionally complete? Few people can make that claim. But that's okay, because over the course of a day or two you probably eat a variety of foods that help you reach a nutritional balance. The same can apply to your cat. Your cat also needs a variety of foods to maintain her health. When you offer your cat a variety of high-quality foods, her nutritional needs will balance out and be met.

Variety

Do you like to eat the exact same thing at every meal, every day of the week? Well, your cat doesn't, either. He wants variety. Variety means just that: Try different meats (including small amounts of organ meats), fowl, fish, and eggs, based on what your cat and can tolerate. Feeding your cat a variety of foods allows him to get the nutritional balance he needs. At the same time, cats can be finicky, especially if they are not feeling well. Therefore it's important to have a few recipes that your cat likes so you can rotate them for variety or if you need to make a switch because he decides he isn't going to eat a certain food one day.

RECIPES

Here are a variety of recipes you can prepare for your cat. When looking for cat food recipes, be sure to choose those that have been prepared by an expert in feline nutrition or a veterinarian who has knowledge of feline dietary needs. You will find lots of recipes on the Internet and in books that have been prepared by well-meaning individuals that may not necessarily be nutritious for your cat. When in doubt about any recipe, consult an expert.

Here are two recipes courtesy of Dr. Cathy Alinovi and Susan Thixton, from *Dinner PAWsible*. Each recipe will feed one 10-pound cat for one day, divided into two meals. Simply combine all the ingredients and store covered in the refrigerator until ready to use. If you double or triple the recipe, be sure to freeze any portions you do not plan to use within 2 to 3 days.

Recipe #1

½ cup shredded or ground cooked turkey breast
   without the skin
2 Tbs chicken hearts, cooked and ground
1 tsp black beans, mashed
1 tsp cod liver oil
150 mg calcium carbonate or slightly less than ⅛ tsp
   powdered eggshell

Recipe #2

½ cup shredded or ground cooked turkey breast
    without the skin
2 Tbs chicken liver, cooked and ground
3 medium-large shrimp (or 4–5 salad shrimp), no
    tails, chopped
1 Tbs red beans, mashed
1 tsp cod liver oil
150 mg calcium carbonate or slightly less than ⅛ tsp
    powdered eggshell

The following two recipes are variations on meals
provided by veterinarians.

Recipe #3

1 lb ground beef
1 cup chicken gizzards, chopped
½ cup sweet peas, frozen or canned (no salt)
1 tsp flaxseed, ground
1 Tbs salmon or fish oil
1 egg, beaten
1 tsp calcium carbonate supplement

Combine the beef, gizzards, and peas in a large sauce
pan and add just enough water to cover all the ingredients. Cover and simmer until the beef is nearly done.
Then add the remaining ingredients, stirring for several minutes until the egg is done and well distributed.
A serving size is ½ cup. You can freeze this recipe in
a cupcake tin.

Recipe #4

⅔ cup mashed sweet potatoes, white potatoes, or
    cooked barley
1⅓ cups chopped cooked turkey or salmon

4 Tbs cooked chicken liver, mashed
4 tsp fish or salmon oil
1 tsp iodized salt
450 mg calcium carbonate

Combine all ingredients and mix well. Divide into six servings, enough for one 10-to-12-pound cat for three days.

PART II

Feline Conditions and Home Remedies

Before you explore any of the chapters in this section, here is a brief explanation of what you can expect to find in the following pages. These points are offered to help you and your cat get the most benefit from the information.

#1. The cat health problems in the following chapters were chosen based on several criteria; namely, (1) they are among the most common disorders or conditions among cats; (2) it's easy to treat these conditions with home remedies such as dietary changes, nutritional supplements, and herbal remedies; (3) the selected remedies have shown some scientific and/or widespread anecdotal evidence they may be beneficial; and (4) the remedies are readily available for consumers. The size and scope of this book limit the amount of useful information that can be covered in a comprehensive manner. Therefore, if you do not see a specific symptom, ailment, or disease in this book, that does not mean it cannot be managed or treated with home remedies. As always, you should consult your veterinarian or feline nutritionist about any concerns or questions, and you can also seek additional information with the help of sources listed in the Appendix or other sources offered by professionals.

#2. Consult a professional veterinarian and get a diagnosis before you start home treatment. If you are well prepared when you make the phone call—if you've noted your cat's signs and symptoms and other information—you can significantly help your veterinarian with the diagnosis. The information in these chapters can help you be prepared as your cat's health advocate.

#3. When choosing new foods, nutritional supplements, or herbal remedies for your cat, consider these tips:

- **Get the supplement in a form your cat will take.** Cats are naturally suspicious and cautious, especially when they "know" you are trying to give them something new in their food or as a supplement. The remedy or supplement needs to taste good and be in a form she will accept. Chewable tablets, powders, and liquids that can be added to food are preferable to pills and capsules.

- **Remedies and supplements should not interfere with any other treatments you are giving your cat.** Ask your veterinarian if the remedies or supplements could interact negatively with other medications or supplements your cat may be taking.

- **Determine the safest and most effective dosage of the supplement or remedy for your cat.** Many recommended dosages for cats are based on veterinarians' experiences, not on scientific or clinical studies, and each cat's needs are different. Therefore, consult a professional before initiating home remedies.

- **Home remedies should be convenient and cost-effective.** If not, you will be less likely to continue treatment as long as necessary. However, also keep in mind that the supplement may prevent or eliminate a symptom or disease, which in turn could prevent costly veterinary bills down the road. If a supplement or remedy is available in a pill or capsule and these forms are more inexpensive than liquid or powders, ask a professional whether you can crush the pills or open up the capsules to deliver the remedy to your cat.

- **Don't give your cat supplements or remedies designed for people unless you first consult your veterinarian about the exact product you want to use.** Not only are dosages for cats and people different, but supplements made for you may contain extra ingredients that could prove harmful to your cat.

#4. When I talk about studies, there are some terms you should know. "Randomized" means the study subjects were randomly assigned to their groups. A "controlled" study means there was a group in the study that did not receive the active ingredient. For example, one group of cats may have been given an herbal remedy, while the control group was given a placebo. "Double-blind" means neither the study's authors nor the vets and/or pet parents knew which cats were getting the active ingredient in the study (e.g., the herb, supplement, or nutrient).

#5. Each chapter provides the top three or more effective and commonly used home remedies for each condition. If there are other supplements or remedies that may have some merit, they are listed separately under "Other Home Remedies," with a brief explanation of each.

Chapter 4
Allergic Dermatitis

"Allergic dermatitis" is a general term that describes a variety of allergies that can affect your cat through the skin. An allergy is the immune system's reaction to a substance (allergen) that the body identifies as foreign. Because the body does not want this foreign substance, the immune system produces a protein called immunoglobulin E, which attaches itself to mast cells in the skin. The joining of immunoglobulin E and the mast cells causes the release of chemicals called histamine. In cats, this sequence of events and substances occurs only within the skin, regardless of what the cat is allergic to.

Therefore, if your cat is allergic to chicken, he will scratch and have other signs and symptoms of allergic dermatitis whenever he eats food that contains chicken. If he is allergic to bee stings and is stung by a honeybee, he will have itching sensations all over his body and may develop skin lesions. Among cats, the skin is the organ that responds to allergens, which may be why so many cats suffer with allergic dermatitis.

DOES MY CAT HAVE ALLERGIC DERMATITIS?

"My cat used to wear a collar with a little bell on it, and she was scratching her neck so much, I took her collar off because the jingling bell was driving me crazy. And I feel so bad for her!" Does this sound familiar? In addition to persistent scratching, especially of the neck, top of the head and ears, lower chest, and belly, cats with allergic dermatitis typically display the following signs and symptoms:

- Licking, chewing, or biting the feet, ears, and skin, which can result in skin lesions. Such lesions can be small to large areas that can bleed and ooze, resulting in a secondary bacterial infection.
- Pulling out tufts of hair
- Crusty scabs, pus-filled bumps, or other bumps on the skin
- Patches of hair loss
- Twitchy skin
- Increased skin pigmentation
- Shaking of the head
- Thickened skin
- Swollen eyelids (typically with food allergies)
- Inflamed, red ears with a moist discharge (with food allergies).

TYPES AND CAUSES OF ALLERGIC DERMATITIS

Three main types of allergic dermatitis are seen in cats:

- **Atopy,** which is an allergic condition caused by inhaling allergens or allergens that are absorbed through the skin. This type of allergic dermatitis is usually seen in young adult cats. The allergens could be anything ranging from pollen to mold, dust, and grasses, or it may be associated with items in the house, such as floor polish, rug cleaner, or detergents. Did you recently get a new upholstered chair that your cat lies on? Your cat could be reacting to chemicals used in the fabric. Some cats are more susceptible to developing certain allergies because of genetic factors, while allergic signs may be related to seasonal changes.
- **Flea bite allergy,** which also affects young adults most often. Fleas and mites are a significant problem for cats, and therefore they are discussed separately in chapter 11.

- **Food allergy (food hypersensitivity),** which can affect cats of any age. The most common allergens for cats are beef and milk products, wheat, corn, soy, chicken, and eggs. Symptoms can appear at any age, whether your cat has been eating the same diet for years or you recently introduced a new food. Ear infections sometimes accompany food allergy symptoms.

Cats may also have a reaction to medications or to parasites other than fleas (e.g., mites, ticks, and intestinal worms), or they may develop skin problems associated with hormones or bacteria. Unfortunately, it is possible for your cat to have more than one type of allergic dermatitis, which also makes it more difficult to diagnose.

DIAGNOSIS OF ALLERGIC DERMATITIS

When you bring kitty to the veterinarian, a variety of diagnostic tests could be ordered once the doctor has conducted a history and physical examination. Those may include:

- Scraping of the skin
- Skin cytology
- Complete blood count and biochemical profile
- Intradermal allergy testing
- Allergy blood tests
- Dietary trials (elimination diet) to identify food allergies.

A diagnosis of atopy is made through a process of elimination: that is, by ruling out other causes such as fleas, mites, bacterial and yeast infections, and food allergies. At that point, the veterinarian may suggest various skin or blood testing for different allergens to help identify the cause of the itching and scratching. If you discover that your cat has atopy, you should know it is a chronic condition with no known cure, but it can be managed using home remedies alone or a combination of conventional and home treatments.

To diagnose a food allergy, your cat can be put on an elimination diet for eight to twelve weeks, during which time he will eat a protein source he has not had previously. This can be a good time to try a homemade diet. (See "Home Remedies" on page 66.) If your cat has a food allergy, you should notice a significant improvement in his symptoms during the trial period. To identify all the foods that bother your cat, your veterinarian will recommend you add a single protein (e.g., fish) back into your cat's diet every one to two weeks and wait to see how your cat reacts.

Diagnosis of flea allergy dermatitis, which is actually a hypersensitivity to flea saliva, is diagnosed by looking for usual signs of fleas (including fleas and flea dirt), skin sores, and scratching. Since flea allergic dermatitis can look like other conditions, your veterinarian may do a skin test to confirm that fleas are the problem.

CONVENTIONAL TREATMENT

Treatment of allergic dermatitis depends on the type of allergy your cat has. The number one treatment is avoiding the culprit allergen(s), if this is possible. If you learn that Winston, your seven-year-old tabby, is allergic to the carpet cleaner you have been using, then a product change and perhaps something to soothe the itch until the allergen is removed from Winston's environment is all that's needed. Helping your cat avoid other allergens might not be so easy, especially if the offending allergens are readily available in your neighborhood.

Topical products that can relieve itching include anti-itch and antibacterial shampoos, antihistamines, topical anti-inflammatory and antibacterial drugs, and corticosteroid therapy, such as hydrocortisone sprays and ointments. The problem with topical medications is that cats will lick them off unless you put a cone collar on your cat or the medication is used on top of the head, on the ears, or under the chin.

Some pet parents choose allergy shots (immunotherapy) to relieve symptoms. The effectiveness of this series of injections varies, although allergy shots reportedly provide at least some relief for about 75 percent of cats with atopy. Pet parents can be taught how to give the injections.

Cats who have scratched themselves excessively may develop bacterial skin infections, which will need treatment with antibiotics. If food is suspected as the cause of allergic dermatitis, an elimination diet may be tried. (See "Home Remedies" on page 66.)

Here are some of the medications your veterinarian may recommend for treatment of allergic dermatitis.

- **Antihistamines.** Most of the antihistamines used for cats are the same ones used for people. However, you should not give your cat your antihistamines without first consulting your veterinarian. Antihistamines can be effective in controlling allergic symptoms in up to 70 percent of cats. If you combine antihistamines with home remedies, you can get even better results. Each antihistamine has a different dose and risk of side effects and should not be used without first consulting your veterinarian. Antihistamines typically come in two forms: H1 and H2 blockers. Those in the latter category include cimetidine and have an effect on the gastrointestinal track. H1 blockers, such as cetirizine (Zyrtec), have been studied in cats who have allergic skin disease and the results have been positive. Other H1 blockers include diphenhydramine (similar to Benadryl), loratadine (Claritin), and chlorpheniramine (Chlor-Trimeton). Possible side effects include dry mouth, nausea and vomiting, drowsiness (less likely with cetirizine and loratadine), and breathing difficulties.

- **Corticosteroids.** Also referred to as steroids, these drugs can be very effective in relieving severe itching and inflammation, but the potential side effects can be serious. Steroids can be given to your cat either by mouth or injection. Injectables include betamethasone, dexamethasone, flumethasone, methylprednisolone, and triamcinolone. It is easier to customize oral dosing and therefore better control any side effects that may occur. They may include increased water consumption, increased urination, weight gain (increase in appetite), depression, and diarrhea. Long-term use of steroids can cause permanent, severe harm, including liver damage, diabetes, adrenal suppression, and an increased risk of infections. A 2012 study in *Veterinary Dermatology* reported that a comparison of triamcinolone and methylprednisolone for treatment of allergic dermatitis in cats found triamcinolone to be seven times more potent than methylprednisolone and that both drugs were well tolerated and effective.

- **Cyclosporine.** This is an immunosuppressant, which means it reduces the response of the immune system to allergens. Cyclosporine is used in dogs for atopy but off-label in cats. It can take three to four weeks before you see any benefit from cyclosporine, and there is the possibility of side effects. A 2012 study, for example, reported on fifty cats treated for allergic dermatitis with cyclosporine. Sixty-six percent of the cats experienced adverse effects, with vomiting or diarrhea being the most common (24 percent), followed by weight loss (16 percent), weight gain (14 percent), and gingivitis (10 percent).

HOME REMEDIES

The home remedies for allergic dermatitis depend in part on the cause of the problem, which needs to be addressed first.

If your cat has fleas, then chapter 11, "Fleas," can be helpful. If your kitty has atopy or food allergies, then reducing or eliminating the allergens from your cat's environment and/ or diet are critical.

In all cases, however, what remains is a cat who is suffering with itchy skin and other skin irritations and problems that can be addressed using home remedies. If necessary, these home remedies can be used along with conventional medications your veterinarian may have recommended.

Apple Cider Vinegar

For cats with flea bite dermatitis, there are two remedies that may be helpful. One is equal parts apple cider vinegar and water. Use it at room temperature or slightly cooled (especially if the weather is hot) and put in a spritzer bottle. Spritz the mixture onto your cat's fur and then work it into the fur and skin.

An oral combination of apple cider vinegar and honey may also provide some relief. Mix ¼ teaspoon of honey and apple cider vinegar and use an eyedropper to add it to her food twice a day.

German Chamomile and Tea

If your kitty has "hot spots" where he has scratched until his skin is red, oozing, and hairless, there are two things you should do. First, allow the areas to dry out (matted hair over the area can lead to infection), which may mean you need to shave or clip the hair around the affected spots. You may need to put an Elizabethan collar on your cat to allow the hot spots to air out. Then gently clean the hot spots with a combination of German chamomile extract and warm water: 15 drops of extract in 4 ounces of warm water, two to three times a day. In addition, apply a cool compress of black or green-tea tea bags to the hot spots two to four times daily.

Marigold Ointment

The common flower, the pot marigold (*Calendula officinales*), has a natural ability to soothe itchiness. You can make your own marigold ointment to apply to your cat's hot spots. After you have allowed the hot spots to dry out (see "German Chamomile and Tea" above), treat the areas with marigold ointment. Here's the recipe to make your own ointment:

    2 oz dried marigold flowers
    2 oz cooking oil
    10 fl oz melted cocoa butter

Put half the flowers into the inside pan of double boiler and pour in the oil and butter. Half fill the outer pan with water. Bring to a boil, reduce the heat, and simmer for two hours. Keep checking to make sure the water does not boil away. Allow the oil to cool and strain. Then repeat the process using the other half of the flowers using the same oil so the finished product is twice the strength of marigold infused oil. Store in the refrigerator.

Omega-3 Fatty Acids

The omega-3 fatty acids derived from fish, which include EPA and DHA, can help reduce the level and effects of histamine and other chemicals your cat's body releases in response to allergens. Although not every cat responds to omega-3 fatty acid supplements, many get at least partial relief. If you choose omega-3s, be patient, as it can take up to several months of treatment before you notice a significant improvement.

The good news about omega-3 fatty acids is that they are very safe, have few to no side effects, and can greatly improve the quality of your cat's fur and skin. When omega-3s are used along with conventional medications for allergic dermatitis, use of the drugs can often be significantly reduced or eliminated. A suggested dose of omega-3 (EPA and DHA) is 1,000 mg daily, which can be given in divided doses in her food. Prick a fish oil capsule with a pin and squeeze out the oil.

Watercress

Watercress (*Nasturtium officinale*) has been considered a tonic herb since ancient times, valued for its ability to clear toxins from the body and for purifying the blood. Nasturtium is also known for treating skin problems such as rashes, eczema, infections, and eruptions. To ease the itch and irritation associated with allergic dermatitis, rub nasturtium tincture into the affected area. Do not use on skin that is broken or oozing. In that case, try German chamomile.

Chapter 5

Cognitive Dysfunction Syndrome

Advances in veterinary medicine and natural medicine—along with lots of loving care—have extended the life spans of domesticated cats and allowed pet parents to spend more years with their cats than ever before. Alas, with advancing years often also comes a decline in various bodily functions, including vision, hearing, mobility, and kidneys. One area of functional decline that is gradually getting more attention—fortunately—is cognitive functioning. In other words, more and more cats are experiencing signs and symptoms of dementia—kitty Alzheimer's if you will—also known as cognitive dysfunction syndrome.

According to a 2011 article in *Topics in Companion Animal Medicine*, about one-third of cats aged eleven to fourteen years develop at least one "geriatric" behavior, such as crying loudly at night or wandering, and this number increases to more than 50 percent among cats fifteen years and older. While some behavior changes in older cats can be attributed to physical health problems, degenerative changes also occur in the brain.

Melissa Bain, DVM, diplomate of the American College of Veterinary Behaviorists, has noted that up to 40 percent of cats older than seventeen years old can demonstrate signs of severe impairment in their cognitive abilities. Little research has been conducted thus far on cognitive problems in cats. In fact, dogs have an advantage in this area, as there has been some significant research into cognitive dysfunction syndrome in dogs, with treatments identified as well. The same cannot be said for cats, but experts have learned that cats do develop behavior changes as they get older, and that some of what has been learned about dogs and cognitive problems can be applied to cats.

That said, it can be a challenge for pet parents and veterinarians to manage the geriatric population of kitties. The good news, however, is that research done in dogs has provided some useful information, and there are steps you can take to help your cat enjoy her golden years. That journey begins with an understanding of cognitive dysfunction syndrome in cats.

DOES MY CAT HAVE COGNITIVE DYSFUNCTION SYNDROME?

Simone is a sixteen-year-old Persian mix who started causing quite a stir in the neighborhood when she began crying loudly at the windows in the middle of the night. "My neighbors thought I had a baby," said pet parent Barbara, who was losing sleep because of the noise. "I explained to everyone that, no, I was not babysitting my grandchild overnight, that the crying was Simone. She has always been a healthy cat, and when I took her to the vet clinic, they couldn't find anything wrong physically. When we started to discuss the signs of cognitive dysfunction, however, then the pieces fell into place."

Simone had also begun to display another behavior that is in fact the most common one associated with cognitive dysfunction: inappropriate elimination, which for most pet parents means their cat no longer uses the litter box or uses it only occasionally. This includes problems with both urination and defecation. It's important to remember that cats with cognitive problems who are not using the litter box are doing it not to be mean or because they are mad at you but because of brain changes. Other signs of cognitive dysfunction syndrome in cats may include:

- Sleep-wake cycle changes (e.g., your cat is agitated at night and sleeps all day)

- Wandering, pacing, and/or reduced activity
- Spatial disorientation, such as walking into corners and standing there as if forgetting where to go
- Changed behavior with pet parents and other pets in the house, which may include seeking increased attention or aggression/irritability
- Reduced grooming
- Excessive licking behavior
- Reduced or lack of interest in food or, less often, more interest in food, which may actually be forgetting they have just been fed.

CAUSES OF COGNITIVE DYSFUNCTION SYNDROME

It's become obvious to researchers that some of our aging feline friends can suffer with a reduction in their ability to think clearly and to remember things like "Hey, where's the litter box?" Thus cats can suffer with age-related deterioration of mental ability, resulting in dementia much like people what people develop. Although the exact cause of this cognitive decline is still a puzzle, just it is in humans, experts have indicated that deterioration of blood flow to the brain, chronic free radical damage (which can destroy healthy cells in the brain), blood vessel changes with age that result in reduced blood flow, and hardening of the arteries (arteriosclerosis) are possible explanations for a decline in cognitive function in cats. Another possibility is the same one that occurs in humans, which is the accumulation of certain type of protein (e.g., tau and beta-amyloid) in the brain, which impairs the ability of the brain to function effectively. Since cognitive decline typically occurs in older cats, confounding factors can be other health problems often seen in elderly kitties, such as heart disease, high blood pressure, and anemia.

DIAGNOSING COGNITIVE DYSFUNCTION SYNDROME

If you have an older cat who is beginning to show signs of cognitive problems, then it may be time to have "the talk" with your veterinarian to discuss signs and symptoms of mental decline. Your veterinarian will rely a great deal on your input when making a diagnosis, so it's important that you accurately describe any unusual behaviors your cat may be displaying, including when the behaviors started, how they have progressed, and when new ones started.

Currently there are no tests that can diagnose cognitive dysfunction in cats; therefore your veterinarian will need to make the diagnosis by excluding other possible causes of your cat's behaviors. Possible factors can include arthritis (the discomfort and pain of arthritis is often underrecognized in older cats), diabetes, high blood pressure, urinary tract infection, gastrointestinal disease, neurological disorders, kidney disease, liver disease, feline immunodeficiency virus (FIV), hearing and/or visual impairments, and feline leukemia, all of which may be mistaken for cognitive dysfunction. Cognitive dysfunction syndrome can exist along with any of these health problems as well.

To make a diagnosis, veterinarians typically

- ✓ Conduct a complete physical examination, including taking blood pressure, as hypertension is common in older cats and can cause signs and symptoms of cognitive dysfunction syndrome
- ✓ Take a full medical history, including use of medications
- ✓ Ask about any exposures to toxins, drugs, and trauma
- ✓ Inquire about behavioral changes and any recent changes to the cat's environment
- ✓ Conduct blood tests, including thyroid hormone levels
- ✓ Take a urine sample for urinalysis

✓ Test for feline leukemia, feline infectious peritonitis (FIP), feline leukemia virus (FeLV) if there is reason to believe these infections are a possibility

✓ Order computed tomography or magnetic resonance imaging of the head if there has been trauma or there is suspicion of a brain tumor.

CONVENTIONAL TREATMENT

Some of the scientific efforts to prevent dementia and memory loss in people also involve our companion animals, and so there are a growing number of drug options for cats who have cognitive dysfunction syndrome, even though none of these medications have been specifically approved for this purpose. You will find considerable anecdotal evidence, however, of how a number of pharmaceuticals used to treat dogs with cognitive dysfunction may also benefit cats.

For example, the drug selegiline (Selgian, Anipryl), which is also used in people for dementia but under different brand names, has been used successfully in dogs who have cognitive dysfunction syndrome. Selegiline increases the concentration of a brain chemical called dopamine, which is involved in cognitive processing.

For now, the research involving the use of selegiline in cats is very limited, but some veterinarians prescribe it because there are anecdotal reports of success. In fact, the American Association of Feline Practitioners supports the use of selegiline for the treatment of cognitive dysfunction syndrome in cats.

Other drugs that may be prescribed by your veterinarian to help with signs and symptoms of cognitive dysfunction syndrome include the following. Never give any of these drugs to your cat without guidance from your veterinarian, as they can be toxic if dosing is not followed carefully.

• **Buspirone.** The antidepressant drug buspirone is sometimes prescribed for cats to help manage behavior problems and to reduce anxiety and fear. These properties make buspirone a good candidate for some cats who are experiencing these symptoms as part of cognitive dysfunction syndrome. The typical dosage for cats is 5 mg twice daily, although your veterinarian will determine the safest dose for your cat. Buspirone is not safe for cats who have kidney or liver disease. Possible side effects include an increase in playfulness, which for many pet parents is a good effect of the drug. However, the drug may also cause an increase in agitation or aggression.

- **Diazepam (Valium).** Diazepam is a benzodiazepine, a class of sedatives that work by reducing levels of certain chemicals (e.g., serotonin, acetylcholine) in the brain. It is sometimes prescribed for cats who are suffering with anxiety as part of cognitive dysfunction syndrome. A typical oral dose can range from 1 to 4 mg every twelve to twenty-four hours. Although diazepam is not approved by the FDA for use in pets, veterinarians are allowed to prescribe it for off-label use. Side effects may include weakness, problems with coordination, and, in some cats, agitation. Although rare, severe, often fatal liver problems develop in some cats who take diazepam.

- **Fluoxetine (Prozac).** Although commonly prescribed for people, fluoxetine is frequently recommended for cats who are experiencing behavior problems, such as aggression or spraying. Sometimes referred to as puppy Prozac, this antidepressant increases levels of serotonin in the brain. A typical oral dose for cats is 2 to 5 mg daily. Side effects may include aggression, excessive vocalization, hyperactivity, loss of appetite (temporary), panting, restlessness, and tremors.

- **Nicergoline (Fitergol).** Nicergoline is a drug used that blocks brain chemicals associated with memory problems (e.g., serotonin, and dopamine). This drug can block serotonin and dopamine receptors and promote blood flow to the brain, which in turn may improve cognition. Use of nicergoline in dogs has resulted in an improvement in activity, mood, and coordination.

- **Propentofylline (Vivitonin).** This is typically given to older dogs to help improve confusion, excessive barking, lethargy, and breathlessness. The drug works by improving the delivery of oxygen to the body, including the brain.

HOME REMEDIES

Home remedies for cats who are living with cognitive dysfunction syndrome are mainly concerned with nurturing and supporting a good quality of life, which includes natural supplementation as well as allowing you and your cat to spend quality time together. Here are some suggestions.

Diet

Studies indicate that older cats who are fed a diet supplemented with antioxidants and essential fatty acids live longer, are more healthy, and display an improvement in cognitive function and mobility than cats who did not receive the supplements. However, changing the diet of a cat who is already experiencing signs and symptoms of memory and cognitive problems may be a challenge, depending on the extent of the modifications. Naturally, if your aging cat refuses to accept a new diet, then you must allow her to eat what she likes. However, gradual, incremental changes can be accomplished. Slow introduction of homemade foods, such as those discussed in chapter 3, are recommended, along with the supplements suggested below.

Antioxidants

Because cognitive problems are associated at least partially with free-radical damage to brain cells, supplementing your cat's diet with antioxidants may help ward off or slow down some of this damage. Dietary supplements for cats that contain vitamins C and E, selenium, flavonoids, and carotenoids (especially beta-carotene) may help put a little more bounce into your cat's declining years. It is best to choose antioxidant supplements especially formulated for cats, as they are typically in a form that you can sprinkle or pour on your cat's food. Do *not* select antioxidant formulas that are for dogs and/or that contain alpha-lipoic acid, a powerful antioxidant that is toxic in cats.

Thus far, researchers have not done many studies concerning the potential benefits of giving antioxidants to cats who have cognitive dysfunction syndrome. However, one five-year study looked at the impact of feeding a branded diet supplemented with vitamin E, beta-carotene, omega-3 and omega-6, and dried whole chicory root (which is supposed to support bacteria in the intestinal tract) for cats age seven years and older. The results of this study showed that cats who were fed the supplemented food lived significantly longer and in better health than cats not given the supplemented food. Note that this study was conducted by the manufacturer of the food, so the results could be skewed. However, studies in dogs have shown antioxidants to provide some benefit for cognitive function, including a 2012 study in which a diet rich in antioxidants improved and maintained cognition in beagles as well as reduced damage to cells from free radicals. Other specially supplemented cat foods also have been shown to help cats who have cognitive dysfunction syndrome. Therefore, can adding antioxidants to your cat's diet hurt? Probably not, and it very well could help and is worth a try.

Choline

Choline is a member of the B vitamin family and a phospholipid, a type of lipid that is part of the composition of cell membranes. Benefits of choline include promotion of healthy cell membranes, support of the nervous system, and helping cats who experience symptoms of cognitive dysfunction syndrome. An over-the-counter product called Cholodin-FEL contains choline as well as another common phospholipid, phosphatidylcholine, and various nutrients, including taurine. Choline and phosphatidylcholine are precursors (instigators, if you will) to brain chemicals called neurotransmitters, which are responsible for sending signals and messages in the brain.

Because choline (Cholodin-FEL) increases brain activity, possible side effects of the supplement include hyperactivity (dashing around the house, climbing activity, howling), muscle twitching, and, in rare cases, aggression. All of these side effects can be corrected by stopping the supplement for several days and then restarting it at a lower dose. If you prefer to bypass Cholodin-FEL and give your cat choline supplements only, consult your veterinarian for the proper dose.

L-carnitine

L-carnitine is an amino acid that has been shown to possibly help individuals who have early-onset Alzheimer's disease. Unfortunately, scientific studies to support the use of L-carnitine in cats with mental challenges are lacking. However, results of several studies of dogs who were given L-carnitine have often suggested the supplement can improve cognitive functioning. The benefit may come from the ability of L-carnitine to enhance mitochondrial function. The mitochondria are organelles in all cells that are essential for energy production. Healthy mitochondrial function is believed to be necessary for brain cell function. If you want to give your cat an L-carnitine supplement, discuss the appropriate dose with your veterinarian. Possible side effects include nausea, vomiting, and loose stools.

Omega-3 Fatty Acids

Admittedly the research showing how omega-3 fatty acids can improve an aging cat's ability to think and remember better is nearly nonexistent, but there is some limited evidence that the essential fatty acid can benefit dogs who have the same mental decline and also research showing that a deficiency of omega-3s is associated with cognitive decline. So if we assume that what's good for the goose (dog, human) is good for the gander (cat), supplementing cats with omega-3 fatty acids to support brain function may be beneficial. Typically supplements are sold as 1,000 mg gel capsules of omega-3 acids as fish oil (eicosapentaenoic acid [EPA] and docosahexaenoic acid [DHA]) that provide 180 mg EPA and 120 mg DHA. To help manage cognitive problems, you may want to increase this dose, but first consult your veterinarian.

SAM-e

The naturally occurring sulfur compound known as S-adenosylmethionine (SAM-e) is present in every tissue in the body and is involved in a wide range of important processes in the immune system, brain, and elsewhere throughout the body. Scores of studies show SAM-e can be beneficial in the management of arthritis, depression, and liver disease, and in pets, it has demonstrated an ability to help with cognitive function, perhaps because of it works with various B vitamins and interacts with brain chemicals such as serotonin, dopamine, and melatonin.

In any case, a study published in the *International Journal of Applied Research in Veterinary Medicine* in 2012 reported that tablets containing SAM-e improved executive function in older dogs and cats. Executive function is the ability to organize thoughts, focus attention, control impulses, and be persistent. Although the study evaluated both cats and dogs, I will report on the cats only.

A total of sixteen cats aged 8.4 to 13.9 years were studied. Administrators gave the cats cognitive tests and then entered them into the treatment portion of the trial, when the cats were given 100 mg SAM-e or placebo daily for fifteen days. After that time they were tested again. Cats who took SAM-e showed potential improvements in executive function but not in short- or long-term memory. In a previous study of dogs alone, those who took SAM-e improved in their levels of activity and awareness when compared with dogs who did not receive SAM-e.

Cats in the study did not experience any side effects. SAM-e is available as a powder and is virtually tasteless, which makes it easy to add to a cat's food.

Other Home Remedies

Here are some simple yet highly effective home comfort remedies for a cat who has signs and symptoms of cognitive dysfunction syndrome. These actions can greatly improve the quality of life for your cat and reduce stress in your life as well, because you'll know you are taking significant steps to help your cat during this difficult stage of life.

- ✓ **Keep your cat's physical environment as predictable as possible.** That means keeping the physical arrangement of your furniture and other household items stable. Now is not the time to rearrange the living room furniture.
- ✓ **Make sure the litter box is easy to access.** If your cat is unable to get into a box that has high sides, get one with lower sides or provide a ramp so she can get inside. Keep more than one litter box available in different areas of the house, and make sure they are clean at all times.
- ✓ **If your cat used to go outside to eliminate, introduce him to litter boxes in the house.** It may take

a while for your cat to get used to the boxes, but as dementia advances, he may forget how to go outside or get lost.

✓ **Close off areas of the house or access to areas where your cat could become stuck.** These may include an unfinished basement, the space between a washing machine and dryer, or crannies under stairwells. Some cats are adept at opening doors to rooms, closets, and cabinets, and then the doors shut behind them, trapping them inside. You may want to put child safety locks on doors that may tempt your cat.

✓ **If your cat has become severely confused, restrict her access to one safe, comfortable area—a single room if possible.** This should be a place where she has everything she needs: comfy bed, toys, scratching posts, a litter box, food, water, and a window (with a safe way to reach the windowsill if she is having difficulty climbing). Some pet parents leave a radio on in the room. Even though your cat may be very confused and need to be in a safe zone, she will still need plenty of human contact every day.

✓ **Consider using a synthetic feline pheromone, which may reduce any anxiety your aging cat may be experiencing.** Use of pheromones (e.g., Feliway) marks a cat's territory and helps her feel safe and secure. Using pheromones is a good option to lessen your cat's anxiety.

Chapter 6
Conjunctivitis

One of the most common eye problems that affects cats is conjunctivitis. Also known as cat pink eye, conjunctivitis is an inflammation of the conjunctiva, which is a thin membrane that covers the outer layer (sclera) of the eyeball and the back of the eyelids. The condition can affect one or both eyes, and it is contagious. Although conjunctivitis is not life threatening, it can jeopardize your cat's vision if left untreated. The infection also can spread to other areas of the eye and result in corneal ulcers, a painful condition in which an open sore develops in the colored portion of the eye. Because conjunctivitis is contagious, you need to keep any affected cats separated from any other cats in your household, or you may end up with more than one case of conjunctivitis.

DOES MY CAT HAVE CONJUNCTIVITIS?

If your cat is pawing at her eye, she may look cute, but this activity also could be a sign that she has conjunctivitis. In fact, one of the classic signs of conjunctivitis in cats is using a paw to scratch the eye in an attempt to relieve itching. However, there are other signs and symptoms you should look for that indicate a cat has pink eye. They include:

- **Redness.** Pink or red eyes is the most obvious sign of conjunctivitis.
- **Squinting.** Difficulty opening one or both eyes can be a sign of conjunctivitis.

- **Swelling.** The conjunctiva can become swollen or inflamed.
- **Watery eyes.** The eye may water more than usual. Watery eyes occur because fluid accumulates in the eye and causes an increase in the number and size of blood vessels, which then results in a "weepy" eye.
- **Light sensitivity.** Your cat may avoid sunlight or brightly lit rooms.
- **Discharge.** The eye may have a discharge that can range from clear to yellow or dark red. Eye infections caused by bacteria, fungi, or viruses usually have a thick yellow or green discharge that causes the eyelid to stick together. Conjunctivitis associated with allergies will have a discharge that is clear and watery.

Conjunctivitis typically is associated with little or no pain. Therefore, if your cat appears to be in pain when you touch the affected eye, the condition may be something other than conjunctivitis. (See "Diagnosing Conjunctivitis" on p. 85.) Your veterinarian can make that determination.

TYPES AND CAUSES OF CONJUNCTIVITIS

Three types of conjunctivitis are found in cats: serous, purulent, and follicular, all of which can be caused by a variety of factors. However, the most common cause of conjunctivitis in cats is feline herpesvirus and the second most common cause is feline chlamydophila disease.

Feline herpesvirus, also known as feline viral rhinotracheitis, is an acute upper respiratory disease caused by the feline herpesvirus type 1 (FHV-1). If your cat contracts FHV-1, he will have it for the rest of his life, so episodes of conjunctivitis may recur. Pet parents can learn to manage FHV-1 and thus conjunctivitis as well. An indepth discussion of feline herpesvirus appears in chapter 10.

Feline chlamydophila disease is caused by the bacterium *Chlamydophila felis*. Within three to seven days of exposure to the bacteria, cats begin to show signs of conjunctivitis, beginning with a watery discharge from one or both eyes. Other signs of the disease soon follow as the discharge changes to a thick yellowish substance. Occasionally cats also experience mild sneezing, a runny nose, and a mild fever that can lead to lethargy and loss of appetite. If the condition is not treated, it can last for six to eight weeks or longer.

Other possible causes of conjunctivitis include mycoplasmal infection; fungal infections (rare); allergies; injuries to the eye (e.g., if your cat gets into a fight and gets her eye scratched); congenital defects, such as blocked tear ducts; scars from previous infections; chemical irritants; and a cat's facial conformation, especially in the Persian cat.

Now let's look at the three types of conjunctivitis in cats.

Serous Conjunctivitis

A mild form of conjunctivitis is serous conjunctivitis in which the conjunctiva is swollen and pinkish. Discharge from the eyes is watery and clear, and occurs when the eyes are irritated by wind, dust, allergens, or cold weather. Serous conjunctivitis can be the first sign of two other common conditions: feline viral respiratory disease or chlamydophila infection. Mild forms of serous conjunctivitis can be treated at home using over-the-counter medications or home remedies. (See "Conventional Treatment" and "Home Remedies" on pages 86 and 87.)

Purulent Conjunctivitis

In some cats, serous conjunctivitis progresses to purulent conjunctivitis, which means thick secretions containing mucus or pus cause a crust to form on the eyelids. This could be caused by a secondary bacterial infection, such as chlamydophila or mycoplasma. Bacteria are usually involved when one eye is involved first and then the problem develops in the other. However, if both eyes have the discharge simultaneously, the herpesvirus or calicivirus are usually involved. In rare cases, a fungal infection is the cause of purulent conjunctivitis. Your veterinarian can make the final determination so the most appropriate treatment can be used.

Follicular Conjunctivitis

In this form of conjunctivitis, the follicles (small mucous glands) on the underside of the nictitating membrane develop a rough surface that irritates the eye and causes the production of a discharge. (The nictitating membrane is the translucent "third membrane" that covers the eye to protect it. In cats, it usually is visible only when they are in ill health.) Possible irritations may include allergens or infective substances. Once the irritating factor has been eliminated, the follicles remain enlarged and keep irritating the eye, resulting in follicular conjunctivitis.

DIAGNOSING CONJUNCTIVITIS

Veterinarians can often diagnose conjunctivitis simply by evaluating a cat's signs and symptoms, reviewing her medical history, and conducting a physical exam. The physical should include an examination of the conjunctiva, the nictitating membranes, and the external eyelids. Since choosing the correct treatment depends on accurately identifying the cause of the conjunctivitis, your veterinarian may order blood tests or cell cultures if he is uncertain of the cause. A few of the other tests your veterinarian could perform include the following:

- Fluorescein staining to look for ulcers or abrasions on the cornea. It involves placing an orange dye (fluorescein) into the eye and using a blue light to look for damage to the cornea.
- Tonometry, a test that measures eye pressure and helps identify glaucoma

- The Schirmer tear test to see if your cat is producing a sufficient amount of tears. Insufficient tear production can damage the eye.
- Biopsy of the conjunctiva.

A diagnosis of purulent conjunctivitis usually can be made after samples from the conjunctival membrane are examined under a microscope, for example. Cats who have ulcers on their cornea typically have feline herpesvirus conjunctivitis.

CONVENTIONAL TREATMENT

If you have more than one cat at home and one has symptoms and signs of conjunctivitis, it is necessary to keep the affected cat separated from any other cats, as conjunctivitis can spread rapidly. Often veterinarians will recommend you treat all cats in a home, even those who do not appear to have conjunctivitis.

Veterinarians typically suggest one of four ways to treat conjunctivitis, although some can be combined: eyedrops, topical creams, oral medication (e.g., antibiotics), or injections. The treatment is dictated by the cause. Giving a cat eyedrops can be a challenge, but oral drugs can be just as effective. Conjunctivitis that is caused by a bacterial infection, such as chlamydia, is usually treated with antibiotics, while a mild case of conjunctivitis caused by environmental irritants can be treated with eye drops and saline solution.

Cats with serous conjunctivitis typically respond to having their affected eyes cleaned with an ophthalmic irrigating solution available over the counter, artificial tears, or a dilute solution of boric acid for ophthalmic use. All of these products are items you would use for yourself for conjunctivitis, and for your cat you may use the same dosing recommendations as those for adults. If your cat does not improve after twenty-four hours, take her to the veterinarian.

If your cat has purulent conjunctivitis, he may respond to

a topical antibiotic medication applied to the surface of the eye several times a day for one week beyond when the condition appears to have cleared up. A common combination antibiotic used for this purpose contains bacitracin, neomycin, and polymyxin. However, if the conjunctivitis is caused by chlamydophila or mycoplasma, your veterinarian may prescribe eyedrops that contain the antibiotics tetracycline or chloramphenicol. Cats who are carrying chlamydophila may be given a prescription for a three-week course of doxycycline or one week of azithromycin.

If a virus is the cause of conjunctivitis, your veterinarian may recommend an antiviral eye medication. Cats who have conjunctivitis caused by feline herpesvirus often experience recurrent episodes and are also repeatedly contagious. It's important to understand that conjunctivitis associated with feline herpesvirus can be treated but it cannot be completely cured. Eyedrops prescribed to fight herpesvirus can include trifluorothymidine (trifluridine) (Viroptic) and vidarabine (Vira-A).

Cats who have follicular conjunctivitis can benefit from a steroid-based eye ointment, which may reduce the size of the follicles and make the eyeball surface smoother. Cats who do not respond to steroid treatment may need to undergo a procedure in which a veterinarian cauterizes (burns off) the follicles.

HOME REMEDIES

One reason conjunctivitis develops is that the immune system is unable to fight off the microorganisms or other agents that cause this eye problem. Home remedies for conjunctivitis can help strengthen your cat's immune system to ward off the causes of conjunctivitis as well as support and nourish eye tissue. Before you treat your cat with a home remedy, consult with your veterinarian.

The following vitamins and other natural nutrients are available individually or in combination products specifically for cats. If you buy the prepared products, use as recommended on the package.

Bilberry

Bilberry (*Vaccinium myrtillus*) extract is derived from fruits that are similar to blueberries and are also known as huckleberries. Bilberries are rich in an antioxidant called anthocyanosides, which are red pigments shown to be helpful in eye and vascular diseases. Anthocyanosides may help improve blood circulation in the blood vessels in the eye as well as strengthen blood vessel walls. The anthocyanosides in bilberries also are attracted to rhodopsin, a photosensitive pigment in the retinal rods that are involved with night vision.

Research has shown bilberries to be helpful in animals with early stages of eye disorders and retinal damage, and in people with eye fatigue. Oral bilberry supplements are available for cats, and a typical dose is 20 to 40 mg daily. Continue to give bilberry extract to your cat for one to two months after the conjunctivitis has cleared.

Chamomile

Chamomile has a centuries-old reputation as a calming herb, but it also has anti-inflammatory properties and an ability to sooth irritated skin. The flowers of this herb are used for remedies, and they contain volatile oils, flavonoids, and lactones that are credited with the inflammation-fighting powers, while polysaccharide ingredients may provide immune system support.

To make a chamomile tea, use 3 tablespoons of tightly packed dried chamomile flowers or 6 tablespoons of tightly packed fresh flowers for every 8 ounces of water. Boil the water, turn it off, and allow the flowers to steep for fifteen to twenty minutes for a strong tea. Let the tea cool before using. Soak a clean cotton ball or swab and carefully wipe your cat's eye from the inner to the outer corners. Be sure to use a new swab for each eye and for each treatment. Repeat treatment up to three times a day.

If you use a chamomile tincture, dilute 5 drops in 20 mL of boiled water and allow it to cool. Repeat the same procedure you would use to treat with the tea.

Lysine

If your cat has conjunctivitis associated with herpesvirus, then lysine may help. This amino acid may be used to attack the herpes virus using a so-called backdoor approach. Here's how it works. Herpesviruses need an amino acid called arginine to reproduce. If you introduce lots of lysine to the virus, it will take up the lysine in favor of arginine, which then suppresses the reproductive ability of the virus. Lysine is an inexpensive natural remedy that is available in most health food stores in both tablet and capsule form. (Hint: Get the capsule, open it up, and mix the amino acid into your cat's food.)

Choose a lysine supplement that does not contain the preservative called propylene glycol, because it can cause serious blood problems in cats. A suggested dose of lysine is 500 mg twice a day for five days when the conjunctivitis is active, then reduced to 250 mg per day for about thirty days after the infection clears. Because herpes virus never goes away, you may need to treat with lysine again if conjunctivitis returns sometime in the future, which is why some experts suggest giving a cat with herpesvirus 250 mg of lysine daily indefinitely.

Eyebright

Just the name of this herbal remedy sounds like it's meant to help with vision problems. Eyebright (*Euphrasia officinalis*) is a herb that is native to Europe and possesses both antibacterial and anti-inflammatory properties. It is so named because it was valued in centuries past for its ability to manage eye problems. The active ingredients in eyebright

appear to be tannins, which have been shown to reduce inflammation. The best way to use eyebright for conjunctivitis
is as a warm compress, but not all cats will tolerate this form
of treatment. However, if your cat is cooperative, it can be
helpful. A warm compress made with an eyebright tea can
help increase blood flow to the eye, relieve redness, and reduce swelling.

To make the tea for the solution, boil 3 ounces of sterile
saline solution and pour it over 1 tablespoon of dried eyebright or one eyebright teabag. Allow the tea to steep for
fifteen to twenty minutes, then strain out the herb if fresh
was used and allow the tea to cool. Moisten a thin white cotton cloth with the tea and place it over your cat's affected
eye. Attempt to hold the compress on the eye as long as possible. Then use a fresh moistened cloth to wipe away any
crusts or debris from the eye. Do not reuse the cloths because
it can reintroduce infection. Apply a compress twice a day.

Rosemary

Rosemary (*Rosmarinus officinalis*) is an herb that has antioxidant powers and also contains several components shown
to have antiseptic and anti-inflammatory properties, including rosmarinic acid and cineole. The herb also has been
shown to speed up healing from abrasions and other surface
irritations. You can make a rosemary tea and use it to bathe
your cat's eyes, as described in "Chamomile" on page 88. To
make rosemary tea, steep 1 teaspoon of dried rosemary in 8
ounces of boiled water, strain, and cool before using.

Other Home Remedies

- **Astragalus.** The herb astragalus (*Astragalus mem-
  branaceus*) is one of the favorites among traditional
  Chinese medicine herbalists. Astragalus is known
  as an adaptogen, which means it is believed to protect the body against physical, emotional, and mental stress. Studies suggest astragalus has antiviral,

antibacterial, and anti-inflammatory properties. To boost the immune system and fight infections, a suggested dose is 6 drops of astragalus extract daily on your cat's food. If you feed your cat twice a day, you can divide the dose.

- **Echinacea.** Echinacea is one of the more popular herbs used for stimulating and boosting the immune system, and it can be especially helpful for fighting viral infections, including respiratory infections in cats. In fact, a July 2012 research article noted that "standardized preparations contain potent and selective antiviral and antimicrobial activities." Echinacea contains several compounds associated with antiviral properties, including caffeic acid, chicoric acid, and echinacin. To help boost your cat's ability to fight conjunctivitis, a suggested dose of echinacea is 15 to 30 drops of tincture twice a day. Do not give echinacea for longer than two consecutive weeks. Echinacea should not be given to cats who have feline leukemia, feline immunodeficiency virus, feline infectious peritonitis, or diabetes.
- **Goldenseal.** Goldenseal (*Hydrastis canadensis*) has a long tradition of use for skin conditions and ulcers, but in more recent years it has gained popularity in managing respiratory tract infections, eye infections, and wounds. Its healing abilities have been attributed to the alkaloids (berberine, berberastine, and hydrastine) in goldenseal dried roots and underground stems, which are used to make liquid extracts, solid extracts, and teas. In cats, a suggested dose to fight infections is 10 to 20 drops of tincture once daily until the infection clears.

Chapter 7
Dental Disease

When was the last time you checked your cat's teeth? Not recently? Never? Well, it's a good idea to regularly ask your feline companion to "open wide," because it's been estimated that up to 85 percent of cats age two years already have the beginnings of dental problems brewing—something called plaque and tartar—accumulating along the gum line, the front line of periodontal disease. Kittens are not immune: The slow march of dental problems can begin in cats younger than one year old as well, and it is not unusual for six-month-old kittens to already show signs of gum inflammation. When dental problems begin at such a young age, they can rapidly progress to irreversible problems.

Similar to children, kittens and cats of all ages need to have their dental health tended to and monitored. Don't wait until your cat stops eating or shows other signs of being ill because of painful dental problems. Untreated dental problems may lead to more serious problems if bacteria from the mouth get into the bloodstream, when they can then damage the heart, liver, and other organs.

Among the most common dental problems your cat may experience are gingivitis and periodontitis, so that is the focus of this chapter. Here's what you should know about these dental challenges and how you can help care for your cat's teeth and gums to prevent them or at least reduce their damage.

A CAT'S TEETH

The sharp tiny teeth kittens use to nibble on your fingers and toes begin to fall out at about age four to six months, and then the permanent teeth push through the gums. Adult cats should have thirty teeth, including four canines, twelve incisors, ten premolars, and four molars. The good news is cats rarely develop cavities. However, they are much more likely to get gum disease and experience an accumulation of plaque and tartar. As in humans, if this plaque is ignored, it combines with saliva and forms tartar, and the next step is gingivitis, which can develop into periodontitis if it is not treated. Therefore, it's important that you learn how to take care of your cat's teeth at home (see "How to Brush Your Cat's Teeth" on page 98) and how to recognize when your cat needs professional help with her teeth.

DOES MY CAT HAVE PERIODONTAL DISEASE?

"I admit I wasn't diligent about Abby's dental health," admitted Carolyn. "We got her from a friend whose wife had died and he couldn't take care of the cat. He told us Abby was all up-to-date on her shots and vet visits, so we didn't even think to check her teeth. After a few weeks, Abby woke me up one morning by standing on my chest and breathing in my face. Her breath was bad, and so I looked into her mouth and noticed tartar buildup. I don't think her teeth had ever been cleaned."

Many pet parents tend to overlook their cats' teeth, and bad breath can be a hint that something undesirable is going on inside their cats' mouths. Here are the signs of dental disease you should watch for regularly. If you already brush or clean your cat's teeth, you will notice these signs. If you haven't ever looked into your cat's mouth, you may be in for a surprise! Not every hint of dental disease occurs in your cat's mouth.

- Loss of appetite
- Weight loss
- Drooling
- Bloody saliva
- Bad breath
- Chewing on one side of the mouth
- Yellow, black, or brown teeth
- Swollen gums
- Red or bleeding gums (may bleed when you press on them)
- Receding gums
- Broken or missing teeth
- Refusing to eat dry food (if you still feed your cat dry food)
- Refusing to play with chew toys once enjoyed
- Rubbing or pawing at her face
- Vomiting undigested food (evidence of inability to chew)
- Poor grooming (because licking is painful)
- Abscesses on the gums

If you notice any of these signs, make an appointment for a dental visit. The sooner your cat is examined and treated, the better chance she has of getting pain relief and warding off more serious dental problems.

Some individual cats and specific breeds seems to be more susceptible to severe periodontal disease. If you have a Maine coon, a Ragdoll, or an Oriental breed such as a Siamese, be especially vigilant. Older cats are more likely to develop periodontal disease than younger animals.

TYPES AND CAUSES OF PERIODONTAL DISEASE

Periodontal disease occurs in two main stages: gingivitis and periodontitis. Gingivitis is the first stage, and if left untreated or improperly managed it can develop into the more serious stage called periodontitis. Let's start with gingivitis.

Gingivitis

Feline gingivitis is the most common dental problem affecting cats. It is characterized by swollen, red, inflamed gums and is caused by the accumulation of plaque along the gum line. Diet is a contributing factor, as a high-carbohydrate diet (e.g., dry cat food) promotes the development of plaque. The plaque forces the gums away from the teeth, which in turn creates tiny sacs or pockets in the gums that become filled with trapped bacteria and food particles. Over time, the gums become infected and inflamed.

Unless the plaque is removed regularly (it forms every twenty-four to thirty-six hours), it mixes with other materials, including calcium phosphate and calcium carbonate. Although plaque is colorless, it turns brown and yellow when it combines with these other substances and develops into tartar (also known as calculus). The accumulation of tartar on a cat's teeth is the main cause of gingivitis.

Fortunately, you can prevent gingivitis in your cat if you make sure she has routine dental care (which includes care at home). Gingivitis can even be reversed with prompt treatment. But if treatment is delayed or ignored, the inflammation and infections can quickly progress to periodontitis.

Periodontitis

When a cat develops periodontitis, the infection has reached the supporting structures of the teeth, which can then result in abscesses of the roots of teeth and even tooth loss. Cats who have periodontitis may have pockets of pus at the base of their teeth. These pockets can be very painful, and it's likely your cat is having difficulty eating if the dental disease has reached this stage. You will also likely notice a strong odor in your cat's breath.

DIAGNOSING PERIODONTAL DISEASE

It's typically not difficult for veterinarians to see when a cat has periodontal disease once they have conducted an examination of the mouth. However, things are not always exactly as they appear. Your cat's gum infections may also be associated with a variety of diseases, such as kidney and liver failure, nutritional deficiencies, immune disorders, feline viral respiratory disease, and feline panleukopenia. Therefore, even though a veterinarian may observe signs of periodontal disease, there may be a reason to look for underlying disease.

That said, veterinarians use several criteria to determine how severe a cat's dental problem is. A physical examination of a cat's mouth is the first step, with an evaluation of the extent of plaque and tartar, the status of the gums, and the depth of any pockets that have formed around the teeth. If you are thinking *Ouch, that must hurt,* you're right, so your kitty will need to be placed under general anesthesia for a thorough examination to be done.

Pocket depth is measured using a calibrated probe. Full-mouth X-rays are usually ordered because the majority of the structure of teeth is below the surface, so veterinarians need to know what's happening under the gum line so they can make a proper diagnosis and choose the appropriate treatment. Your veterinarian may also order a complete blood count, urinalysis, and/or blood chemistries depending on the general health of your cat.

CONVENTIONAL TREATMENT

If your cat has been diagnosed with gingivitis, her teeth will need to be professionally cleaned at the veterinarian's office. Cats must be given anesthesia before a veterinarian can perform the dental work, which will include removing plaque and tartar and polishing the teeth. After you take your cat home, you should follow the dental plan your veterinarian gives you, which will likely include cleaning your cat's teeth at least several times a week, and preferably daily. You may or may not be advised to place your cat on a special dental-care diet to help reduce plaque and tartar and the recurrence of gingivitis. Some veterinarians claim these special foods can be beneficial, while others say they are not.

Cats who have periodontitis require more extensive treatment, and all the work will be done under general anesthesia. Sometimes cats are started on antibiotics several days before dental treatment begins. Following X-rays of the cat's mouth, the veterinarian will need to remove plaque and tartar, cut away any diseased tissue (subgingival curettage) and/or excess gum (gingiva), drain any pus pockets, and pull any damaged teeth. In severe cases, periodontal surgery may be necessary, which involves opening up the gums and reaching deeper structures. Antibiotics may be placed into infected pockets in the gums during treatment. After treatment, additional antibiotics (e.g., amoxicillin clavulanic acid, clindamycin, and cefadroxil) are commonly prescribed for one to two weeks.

In addition to post-treatment antibiotics, cats who have been treated for periodontitis typically are given pain and anti-inflammatory medication and topical medications. This latter group of medications, which can include chlorhexidine (a disinfectant), stannous fluoride, and zinc ascorbate, are usually applied to the cat's teeth on a regular basis, based on your veterinarian's instructions.

HOME REMEDIES

These home remedies can both help prevent dental problems and treat them should your cat develop gingivitis or periodontitis. The most critical preventive step is routine dental care at home. If you are able to care for your cat's teeth on a daily basis or a few times a week, you will be heads and tails ahead of the game when it comes to dental health.

How to Brush Your Cat's Teeth

The best time to familiarize your cat with having her teeth cleaned at home is now, unless he has periodontitis, in which case attempting to clean the teeth would be painful. In such a case, teeth cleaning will need to wait until after you have had your cat treated professionally and healing has begun. However, during the time when your cat's gums are still painful, you can use a natural mouth rinse (see below).

Otherwise, the younger your cat is when teeth cleaning is initiated, the better. If you have a kitten, it's the ideal time to get him accustomed to having your finger and/or a toothbrush in his mouth. If you're thinking *I could never brush my cat's teeth* or *Sammy would never hold still for that!* the best I can say is: Be gentle, patient, and persistent. The rewards for your cat—and your wallet—can be significant if you can support good oral health at home.

If, however, you have a cat who struggles vigorously and absolutely refuses to have his teeth cleaned at home, you may have to accept the fact that he will need to have them cleaned professionally, which requires sedation. You don't want to jeopardize the good relationship you have with your cat over teeth brushing!

Ideally, cleaning your cat's teeth is a two-parent task, but plenty of parents do it themselves. So here goes!

- Sit on the floor or on a bed, because you will need room to restrain your cat comfortably. Hold your cat facing away from you. If your cat likes to kick and squirm, then you may need to place his lower body in a pillowcase.
- Cradle your cat's head in one hand and tilt it back toward your chest.
- Using the fingers of your other hand, gently lift your cat's jowls on one side of her mouth until you can see her teeth and gums. This is for inspection

purposes only, since this is the hand you will use to clean the teeth. Release your cat's jowls.
- Here's the tricky part: Use the index finger and thumb of the hand that is cradling your cat's head to lift the side of your cat's jowls.
- Use the index finger of your other hand to apply light downward pressure to the space between your cat's two lower front teeth. This will allow you space to clean the teeth.
- Using that same hand, start cleaning the teeth either with a cat toothbrush or your finger covered with a finger cot. You may also use a cotton swab wrapped with a piece of gauze.

Don't get discouraged: It will likely take several sessions before your cat becomes more accepting of the tooth cleaning experience. If you introduce your cat to the process in tiny steps each day, eventually you should be able to clean her teeth without much difficulty. If you give your cat lots of praise during each session and reward her with a small treat, such as a piece of cooked or lightly cooked chicken, then she may be more likely to tolerate tooth cleaning. Some pet parents find that using a small amount of tuna juice in the finger cot or on the toothbrush improves their cat's acceptance of the experience.

TOOTHPASTE FOR CATS

Do *not* use toothpaste meant for humans. If you want to use a commercial product, choose a toothpaste specially made for cats. It is recommended you look for toothpastes that do not contain additives and preservatives, such as xylitol, essential oils, or sugars. Chlorhexidine is an ingredient that can be beneficial, as it can kill plaque above the gum line. If you prefer, you can make your own natural homemade tooth cleaner by using the following ingredients.

(*continued*)

✓ If your cat has gingivitis, combine 30 mg of coenzyme Q10 powder with just enough water, aloe vera gel, or fish oil to make a thin paste. Look for preservative-free aloe vera gel. Use of 30 mg of coenzyme Q10 powder makes enough toothpaste for one cleaning.

✓ For general cleaning purposes, combine 3 tablespoons green tea powder (preferably decaf) and ½ teaspoon vitamin C as calcium ascorbate powder (do not use ascorbic acid) and store the mixture in a tightly sealed glass container. When it's time to clean your cat's teeth, place about 1 teaspoon of the powder mix on a plate and dip a finger cot, cat toothbrush, or piece of gauze in fish oil or water, then into the powder, and then clean the teeth. Your cat may respond better if you use water from a can of tuna (tuna packed in water, not oil) instead of plain water.

Diet

I've already mentioned that a high-carbohydrate diet (i.e., dry cat food) contributes to the formation of plaque because the cat's gums are more sensitive to the bacteria involved in the formation of plaque. Therefore, a dry food diet is a driving force behind the development of gingivitis. However, you have also likely heard that feeding a cat dry food helps to keep the teeth clean. This idea is rapidly losing favor, and even the idea that special dry cat foods are necessary for dental health is disputed by many veterinarians. According to Elizabeth M. Hodgkins, DVM, author of *Your Cat: Simple New Secrets to a Longer, Stronger Life,* "You cannot protect your cat's teeth and gums by feeding 'tartar-control' cat food. Valid clinical trials on 'real' cats over realistic periods of time have not been done to prove that these formulas result in better long-term tooth and gum health in cats." In addition, cats in the wild do not eat dry cat food, nor do they tend to get periodontal disease.

There is also a school of thought that says giving your cat raw chicken bones regularly or a raw-food diet with bones will prevent the development of plaque and tartar. On the other hand, other veterinarians and pet parents are against feeding cats a raw-food diet, including raw bones (cooked ones are too soft and will splinter) because of worries about risk of infection from raw food, ethical reasons (the pet parents', not the cats'), or the "ick" factor. In any case, feeding a cat a raw-food diet and/or occasionally giving a cat raw chicken bones is a personal decision pet parents can make after reviewing the available information and debates and then making their own decision.

More and more veterinarians are beginning to agree, however, that dry food is not good for dental health—or indeed for the overall health—of cats. Therefore, if you want to prevent periodontal disease or help your cat if she already has the disease, feed canned food and/or homemade food.

Natural Mouth Rinses

Several herbal mouth rinses may help your cat's mouth heal. Recommended use is twice a day for about two weeks. Mouth rinses can be administered using a syringe and squirting the rinse into your cat's mouth. Be sure each of these remedies is at room temperature before using them.

- **Echinacea (*E. angustifolia*).** This rinse can be beneficial if your cat has infected gums. Boil 8 ounces of water, add 1 teaspoon fresh echinacea root and allow it to steep for 15 to 20 minutes.
- **Goldenseal (*Hydrastis canadensis*).** This remedy can help promote new gum growth. Boil 16 ounces of water and add 1 teaspoon powdered goldenseal root. Steep for fifteen to twenty minutes.

- **Plantain (*Plantago major*).** If your cat has minor plaque and tartar and inflamed gums, this rinse may help. Boil 8 ounces of water and add 1 table-spoon of plantain leaves. Steep five minutes.

Antioxidants

Two antioxidants may help improve the health of your cat's gums and boost the immune system: vitamin C and vitamin E. Both are very safe for cats and can be added easily to their food. If your cat has gingivitis or periodontitis or is recovering from dental work, a typical daily dose is 100 mg of vitamin C (liquid drops are available) and 200 IUs of vitamin E as natural alpha-tocopherol. Vitamin E is available as a liquid or softgel, which you can pierce with a pin to release the oil. These antioxidants can be given until the symptoms are eliminated.

Chapter 8

Diabetes

Diabetes is not just a people problem; it's a feline challenge, too, and one that is on the upswing. Approximately one in one hundred cats develops diabetes, and it appears that diabetes in cats and in pet parents have some common characteristics. The biggest among them (no pun intended) is obesity. According to Denise Elliott, a medical specialist in nutrition within Banfield's Medical Quality Advancement team, "the evidence clearly demonstrates that obesity from excess calories is the main driver of diabetes mellitus in cats."

If obesity is the main driver, what about the vehicle? I leave that explanation to feline diabetes expert Elizabeth Hodgkins, DVM, author of *Your Cat: Simple New Secrets to a Longer, Stronger Life*, who explains that "diabetes in the cat is a man-made disease, which is completely preventable by avoiding the 'kitty junk-food' that is dry kibbled cat food. Without question, it is the continuous, day-in, day-out consumption of this poor-quality, highly processed, carbohydrate rich 'breakfast cereal for cats' that causes so many felines to become diabetic."

Therefore, this chapter is for every cat parent, whether your cat has diabetes or not, and especially if you have been dishing out "breakfast cereal for cats." Whether you are interested in prevention or treatment, it's time for you to learn more about diabetes in cats.

DOES MY CAT HAVE DIABETES?

Justina is a ten-year-old Persian mix who recently acquired a large appetite and more frequent visits to the litter box to urinate. Her pet parent, Stephen, became concerned because he had a friend whose cat had displayed similar symptoms and the ultimate diagnosis had been diabetes. A visit to Justina's veterinarian for some tests confirmed Stephen's suspicions.

During the early stages of diabetes, cats typically show the same signs as Justina, with an increase in food intake and urination, which is also usually accompanied by increased thirst and water intake. As the disease progresses, other signs and symptoms appear:

- Sweet breath, with an odor like nail polish remover. This is caused by an accumulation of ketones, which are the by-product of the metabolism of fatty acids that form because the body cannot metabolize sugar (glucose).
- Unkempt haircoat
- Loss of appetite
- Weight loss
- Vomiting
- Weakness and lethargy
- Dehydration
- Rapid, labored breathing

TYPES AND CAUSES OF DIABETES IN CATS

Cats who have diabetes are much like people who get diabetes because they usually develop the most common form of the disease: type 2 diabetes. (Dogs, however, get a form of type 1 diabetes.) This means if your cat has diabetes, the beta cells in her pancreas still make some insulin but not enough, or that her body is less sensitive to the insulin it produces. Without enough insulin, your cat's body cannot use glucose properly. Therefore, the sugar accumulates in the bloodstream and leads to increased thirst and increased urination. If not treated properly, diabetes can eventually cause serious, life-threatening complications. Some cats with type 2 diabetes need insulin injections.

Although less common, there are two other types of diabetes that can appear in cats. A much smaller number of cats develop type 1 diabetes, in which cats require daily insulin injections because their pancreases no longer produce any insulin.

The third type of diabetes in cats is called transient diabetes. Cats who have this form of diabetes initially have type 2 disease and need insulin, but over time their system adjusts, allowing them to stop taking insulin. This change typically is related to consuming a high-protein, low-carbohydrate diet. Therefore, if your cat is diagnosed with type 2 diabetes, there is a chance he or she can be cured if a high-protein, low-carbohydrate diet is followed closely.

When the subject of diabetes in cats is raised, the first thing people think of is obesity. Yes, overweight or obese cats are at increased risk for diabetes, because the excess fat makes the cat's body less sensitive to the effects of insulin. Overweight cats are also at risk for other health problems, so pet parents should try to keep their cats at a healthy weight.

Although diet and obesity play significant roles in the development of diabetes in cats, there are several other risk factors to be considered:

- **Age.** Diabetes is more likely to develop in older cats.
- **Chronic pancreatitis.** This is long-standing inflammation of the pancreas.
- **Hyperthyroidism.** See chapter 13 for more on this common condition
- **Medications.** Use of drugs such as corticosteroids and megestrol acetate (Megace) may cause or mimic diabetes in cats.
- **Genetics.** Burmese cats appear to have a genetic predisposition to develop diabetes.

- **Gender.** Male cats are twice as likely to develop
  diabetes as are female cats. Male cats at greatest risk
  are those who are neutered, are older than ten years
  in age, and weigh more than 15 pounds.

Although cats and humans share may characteristics when
it comes to diabetes, cats have an advantage in that they do
not develop atherosclerosis and hypertension along with
their diabetes.

DIAGNOSING DIABETES

In people, diabetes can be diagnosed by taking a blood
sample after a twelve-hour fast and checking the blood glucose levels. In cats, however, the mere act of taking a blood
sample, visiting a veterinarian's office, or being separated
from their pet parent can cause their glucose levels to spike
up to 300 to 400 mg/dL (normal is about 60 to 120 mg/dL),
resulting in a falsely high blood glucose level. Therefore,
veterinarians must rely on more than fasting blood tests to
make a diagnosis: namely, clinical signs and symptoms
(which pet parents can keep notes on to report to their veterinarian) and glycosuria, which is the presence of glucose in
the urine. Clinical signs alone also are not enough for a diagnosis, because both hyperthyroidism and kidney failure, both
of which are common in older cats, have similar signs (see
chapters 13 "Hyperthyroidism," and 15, "Kidney Disease").

Therefore, veterinarians may also use the results of a
fructosamine concentration test to help distinguish stress-
induced high blood sugar (hyperglycemia) from diabetes.
Fructosamine is a sugar-albumin (protein) complex that forms
in cats who have chronic low blood sugar conditions. Fructosamine levels are not affected by stress, which is why vet-
crinarians like to use them in the diagnosis of diabetes in
cats. Other possible clues for diabetes include elevated liver
enzyme levels, high cholesterol, and abnormally low levels
of potassium, sodium, and phosphorus.

CONVENTIONAL TREATMENT

In a 2012 study conducted by the College of Veterinary Medicine at the University of Georgia, Athens, and published in the *Journal of Feline Medicine and Surgery*, surveyed veterinarians revealed how they managed feline diabetics. Of ninety veterinarians who responded to the survey, 74 percent said their clients required chronic insulin, while 26 percent were transient diabetics. Dietary management was recommended by 97 percent of the respondents, with 93 percent of the professionals recommending a prescription or proprietary high-protein, low-carbohydrate diet. The most common cause of poorly controlled sugar levels was mishandling of insulin by pet parents.

Therefore, treatment of diabetes in cats basically involves three strategies: dietary control, medication (usually insulin), and monitoring. I discuss diet under "Home Remedies" on page 109. The good news is that in some cats, the use of insulin (and oral anti-diabetes drugs as well) can be stopped if weight control and a healthy diet are maintained.

Insulin and Oral Antidiabetes Drugs

Most cats with diabetes are managed with insulin. A veterinarian must determine the amount of insulin a cat needs, and this can be done while a cat is hospitalized for a few days after diagnosis so periodic blood samples can be taken to identify her response to the injections. Once an adequate insulin dose is identified, pet parents can be taught how to administer the insulin at home using tiny, extremely thin needles. Most cats with diabetes need one or two insulin injections per day.

The preferred types of insulin for cats are protamine zinc, beef, and pork insulins. Protamine zinc insulin is the only FDA-approved insulin for cats made from recombinant DNA that is identical to human insulin. This insulin is a combination of zinc and protamine, a protein derived from salmon, and has proved beneficial in many cats. Beef insulin is the most similar in molecular structure to insulin in cats, and therefore it is usually the most effective for cats. Pork insulin also is an effective choice.

A cat's insulin needs vary with her diet, so it's important to keep both the amount of calories and the timing of the meals as constant as possible from day to day. It's best to divide a cat's daily ration into smaller meals to help keep sugar levels even. A cat who gets two injections of insulin per day can be given the injections immediately after each feeding. A cat who gets a single insulin injection can be fed her second meal eight to twelve hours after her first meal and the insulin injection, which is when the insulin level should peak. In some cases, an overweight cat with diabetes can be managed by changing the diet alone—no need for insulin!

About one-third of cats with diabetes are treated with oral antidiabetes drugs, at least initially. Options include glipizide and acarbose. Although some cats who start treatment with oral medications may eventually need insulin injections, research also shows that some cats who are taking insulin can be weaned off them after they have switched to oral antidiabetes medication plus a low-carbohydrate diet. In one study from the University of Colorado, for example, cats on a low-carbohydrate diet and who took acarbose were able to reduce their dependence on insulin and also improve control of sugar levels.

Acarbose works by inhibiting the digestive enzymes that metabolize starches, which in turn leads to a more gradual absorption of sugars after your cat eats. You must give acarbose with food if it is to work.

Glipizide works by increasing the secretion of insulin and decreasing insulin resistance, which allows insulin to work on the cells better. Side effects associated with glipizide include diarrhea, flatulence, and constipation, but they can be minimized or eliminated if the drugs are given with food.

The take-home message when it comes to insulin and antidiabetes drug is that it depends on the cat. Some cats require insulin alone, others take both insulin and antidiabetes drugs and can reduce their need for insulin, while others who may have mild diabetes can get along with dietary changes and little or no oral antidiabetes drugs.

Monitoring

You can use a regular "people" glucose monitor to keep track of your cat's glucose levels. Blood samples are usually taken from a cat's ear. An alternative is a commercially available urine testing system that changes color if there is sugar in the urine. A healthy blood glucose level for cats is in the 60 to 120 mg/dL range.

It's important to regularly monitor your cat's glucose levels, because many cats experience periods when the diabetes seems to go into remission, and cats do not need insulin during those times. Giving insulin when it's not needed can result in an insulin overdose, which can become fatal very quickly.

HOME REMEDIES

Some cats who are mildly diabetic may be managed solely with diet and weight control, which means you can avoid use of oral drugs or insulin. However, this approach does not work for every cat, so you should discuss it with your veterinarian. Even if you are not able to control your cat's diabetes with diet alone, modifying her nutrition will go a long way toward improving her quality of life and extending her life span.

Diet

Because cats are carnivores by nature, it's important that your cat get lots of protein and minimal carbohydrates, since a cat's body is not efficient at metabolizing carbohydrates. This is especially true for cats who have diabetes. Feeding your diabetic cat a homemade food diet is recommended, because it allows you to have firsthand knowledge of the ingredients your cat eats. You can, however, choose a high-quality commercial cat food as the only food or alternate homemade recipes with commercial foods.

Is It Dinnertime?

Priscilla the nine-year-old orange tabby was used to snacking anytime she pleased, but after she was diagnosed with diabetes, her pet parent, Karen, had to change that routine. "Now Priscilla gets fed according to her insulin injections," says Karen. "And she wasn't too pleased with the change in routine for a while." Cats who have diabetes should be fed twice a day, with the insulin injection following each feeding. This allows cats to absorb their calories when the insulin is peaking, which prevents them from having low blood sugar (hypoglycemia). Although your schedule may be slightly different, the important part is to be sure your cat has eaten before his insulin dose. If your cat doesn't want to cooperate with the new schedule, you should consult your veterinarian. You may need to return to the grazing schedule for a while and gradually limit when you offer food, and in the meantime adjust the insulin shots to match when your cat is eating the most food. Don't get discouraged!

If you do choose a high-quality commercial cat food, look for those that are high in protein (45 to 70 percent dry matter), moderate in fat (15 to 35 percent dry matter), and low in carbs (0 to 5 percent dry matter), according to Dr. Hodgkins. Much of the dry kibble for cats, however, contains a topsy-turvy breakdown of nutrients: high carbohydrates (35 to 50 percent dry matter from grains), moderate protein (22 to 34 percent dry matter), and low fat (10 to 25 percent dry matter). A discussion on how to determine dry matter in cat food is in chapter 1.

A number of cat food producers have products labeled "for management of diabetes" or similar language. Do not assume, however, that these foods are healthy for your cat. In fact, some of them contain unacceptable amounts of high-carbohydrate ingredients, such as corn in various forms (corn gluten, ground yellow corn, corn flour), rice, and wheat. Be sure to calculate the carbohydrates before you make your purchase, and buy only canned or fresh foods. Another option is homemade foods.

If your cat is overweight or obese, part of your dietary strategy will include weight loss. For maintenance, cats need 20 to 30 calories per pound of ideal body weight per day. Cats who are overweight should be given about 75 percent of their calculated calorie needs. (See chapter 1 for the explanation "How Much Food Does My Cat Need?" on page 28.) Therefore, if your diabetic cat is overweight and should weigh 12 pounds, she needs 180 to 270 calories (75 percent of 240 [20 × 12] and 75 percent of 360 [30 × 12], respectively) of high-protein, very low carbohydrate food per day.

As I explained in chapter 1, the food needs of each cat must be determined on an individual basis. For cats who have diabetes, it is especially important to achieve and maintain a desirable healthy weight, which will help you better manage blood sugar levels and therefore your cat's overall health.

Chromium

Chromium is a mineral that a cat needs in only minute amounts. A well-accepted feature of chromium is that it can enhance the activity of insulin, which in turn has a critical role in the metabolism and storage of carbohydrates, fat, and protein. Taking chromium supplements may help your cat lose body fat (and thus help with obesity), lower blood sugar levels, and reduce cholesterol levels. Most of the studies of chromium and diabetes have been done in humans, but some limited research also has been done in cats.

A University of Queensland study involved thirty-two healthy cats who were randomly assigned to one of four groups: 0, 150, 300, or 600 parts per billion (ppb) of chromium picolinate, an easily absorbed form that combines chromium and picolinic acid. After the cats had taken the supplements for six weeks, those who received 300 and 600 ppb had lower glucose levels than did cats in the other two groups. The researchers suggested cats at risk for obesity and diabetes be given daily supplements of chromium as a preventive measure.

Some pet parents report that chromium supplementation helps in regulating glucose levels in their cats and that it allows insulin to work more effectively and last longer. If you use chromium, it is important to closely watch your cat's blood sugar levels for its effects. A suggested dose is 200 micrograms per day.

A potential side effect of daily supplementation with chromium in a small percentage of cats is an increased risk of kidney disease. In particular, Siamese are at a higher risk for urinary, kidney, and bladder disease and should be monitored closely.

CARING FOR YOUR DIABETIC CAT AT HOME

✓ **If your cat is overweight, help her to lose weight gradually (see Chapter 16, "Obesity").** Cats should not lose more than 2 percent of their body weight per week, or they will be at high risk of liver failure.

✓ **Check your cat's glucose levels at home.** Your veterinarian can show you how.

✓ **Check the litter box regularly to be sure your cat is urinating the same amount.**

✓ **Contact your veterinarian if your cat has any change in her appetite, urine output, water intake, weight, or energy level.**

Other Home Remedies

- **Arginine.** The amino acid arginine should be present in relatively high levels in cats who have diabetes, because it stimulates the beta cells to secret insulin. Fortunately, most meats are high in arginine, but an arginine supplement could further boost the beta cells. Talk to your veterinarian before giving your cat an arginine supplement.

- **Carnitine.** It's known that the amino acid L-carnitine should be present in relatively high levels in the diet of cats who have diabetes and that it helps in transporting fats into cells, which facilitates metabolism and is helpful in cases of diabetes. Exactly how much carnitine to supplement, however, is uncertain.

- **Vitamin E.** Talk to your veterinarian about giving your cat a vitamin E supplement to help with diabetes. Use of vitamin E may help increase circulation and reduce inflammation of the pancreas, which in turn may allow better distribution of nutrients through the bloodstream. You can easily add vitamin E to your cat's food by pricking a hole in a vitamin E gel capsule and squeezing the oil into your cat's food. A dose of 200 IU per day is suggested.

Chapter 9

Ear Mites

Is your kitty scratching her ears so much it's driving you crazy? Imagine how *she* feels! Intense scratching is a signature sign of ear mites in cats. Ear mites (*Otodectes cynotis*) are tiny insects that dwell in the ear canal and feast on the skin and debris that they find there. They are the most common cause of ear infections in cats, and kittens can be infected by their mothers.

All the biting and chewing action done by mites can cause intense itching, which drives cats to scratch both inside and outside the ears. Another type of mite that also affects the ears is the *Demodex cati*, and they are usually found in waxy debris in the ears. These critters like to burrow into the ear, which triggers irritation and an increase in the production of wax.

Just because they are called ear mites doesn't mean these pesky creatures limit themselves to just the ears. Ear mites are known to journey all over a cat's body. In fact, have you noticed how your cat sleeps with the end of his tail tucked up near his ears? That's why cats who have ear mites will also have the pests on their tails. Ear mites also make their way to other cats, dogs, and other house pets, although they do not infect humans.

DOES MY CAT HAVE EAR MITES?

Cats normally scratch their ears from time to time, but when the scratching is persistent and constant, then suspect ear mites. However, other conditions can cause your cat to scratch his ears, so here's a quick (but not foolproof) way to check if your cat has ear mites: Using your thumb and fore-finger, gently massage the back of your cat's ear at the base. Cats who have ear mites usually start to scratch vigorously because you have disturbed the tiny pests. However, cats who do not have ear mites either like the ear massage or try to run away.

Other signs and symptoms of an ear mite infestation include violent head shaking, loss of hair around the ears and/or raw areas and scabs from scratching, and a dry, dark brown, crumbly discharge when you look into your cat's ears. In some cases the discharge may have a foul odor. Some cats flatten their ears back against their head, or they may whimper or cry when scratching if you touch the ears.

Cats with ear mites frequently scratch themselves so much, they damage their ears, causing them to bleed. The tiny breaks in the skin and ears can lead to bacterial infection. If your cat violently shakes her head from time to time, she may cause blood vessels in the ears to break, which can result in the formation of an accumulation of blood outside of the blood vessels (a hematoma).

You can examine the discharge from your cat's ear if you *carefully* remove some of the material that is clearly visible from your cat's ear canal. Do not dig into the canal with a cotton swab or any other object because you may damage your cat's ear. Instead, use a soft cotton cloth slipped over your finger to gently capture the debris. If you have a powerful magnifying glass, you can view the discharge against a black background. You are looking for white specks about the size of the head of pin: These are mites. They may or may not be moving. Dead or alive, you want them gone!

DIAGNOSING EAR MITES

Veterinarians typically diagnose ear mites based on signs and symptoms and by looking into your cat's ears using an otoscope, a lighted magnifying instrument. A microscopic examination of debris and ear wax removed from your cat's ears should identify the culprits. Even if you have already examined the debris from your cat's ears with a magnifying glass or even a microscope, it's best to have a professional diagnosis before beginning treatment, because ear mite medications can cause other problems if they are used when other ear problems are present.

In addition, an accurate diagnosis will allow you to start the right treatment, because ear mites can be serious if left untreated. Ear mites can damage your cat's eardrums, cause secondary bacterial infections, and even result in deafness.

CONVENTIONAL TREATMENT

The first thing you can do for a cat who has ear mites is clip her nails so she won't scratch herself (or you). The next task is to clean her ears. As long as there is excess wax and debris in your cat's ears, ear mites have a safe haven, even if you treat the ears with medications, because the pests can hide in the dirt.

Once your cat's ears are clean, there are a variety of both over-the-counter and prescription medications available to kill ear mites (miticides). Among the OTC medications (e.g., Mita-Clear and Sentry HC Earmite Free for cats) are a number that contain a natural insecticide called pyrethrin, which is often paired with other ingredients such as piperonyl butoxide. These products require that you treat your cat several times, so be sure to follow directions. Prescription medications, including milbemycin oxime (MilbeMite Otic), ivermectin (Acarexx), and selamectin (Revolution) are more toxic than OTC remedies and typically eliminate ear mites from the ears after one treatment, but your veterinarian can advise you best.

Just because you think you killed all the ear mites in your cat's ears doesn't mean you got all of them, since these pests travel all over the body. That means you also may need to treat your cat's entire body with a topical insecticide in the form of a shampoo. Products that are designed to kill fleas and ticks often contain at least one of the above-named ingredients that will kill ear mites on your cat. Be sure to especially shampoo your cat's head and tail, as these are two places mites will hide out. If even one or two mites escape the treatment, they can crawl back into the ear and reinfect your cat. Keep a close eye on your cat, as it can take several weeks before you can be sure your cat is free of mites.

A FEW WORDS ABOUT PYRETHRINS AND PERMETHRIN

Pyrethrins are natural extracts produced from chrysanthemums and are a popular insecticide for cats and dogs. Although there are six different types of pyrethrins (pyrethrin I and II, cinevin I and II, jasmolin I and II), all of which can be found in products for ear mites, fleas, and ticks, manufacturers typically just list "pyrethrin" on their labels.

Pyrethrins work by disrupting the nervous system in insects. The insecticide is often paired with a synergist such as piperonyl butoxide, which enhances the activity of pyrethrins. Side effects caused by cats who ingest pyrethrins are rare, but if they do occur they can include excessive salivation, tremors, vomiting, and seizures. In most cases, however, a cat's stomach acids can break down pyrethrins and not cause a problem, although some pet parents prefer to use completely natural approaches to ear mite control (see "Home Remedies" below).

Pyrethrins can also be combined with permethrin, which is a synthetic pyrethrin. **Because cats are less able to break down permethrin, it is recommended you not use products containing this substance**.

HOME REMEDIES

If you choose to use home remedies to rid your cat of ear mites, you will need to do three steps as you would using a conventional approach, except you can use nontoxic ingredients. Therefore, the first step is to clean your cat's ears, then treat the mites, then treat the entire cat.

Oil and Vitamin E

A combination of oil and vitamin E can be used to clean your cat's ears, but this mixture does a bit more: It helps smother the ear mites and also changes the environment of the ear so the pests are less "happy" staying there.

Combine ½ ounce of almond or olive oil with 400 IU vitamin E (use a pin to prick a hole in a vitamin E gel capsule). Make sure the mixture is around body temperature; that is, it should not be refrigerated or hot. Using an eyedropper, place about ½ dropperful in your cat's ear and gently massage the base of the ear for about a minute so the oil is distributed into the ear canal and releases the debris. Let your cat shake her head—she'll be ready! Use a thin, clean cotton cloth on your finger or a cotton ball to clean out the ear opening, but don't dig into the ear.

Repeat this procedure in the other ear and apply this treatment every other day for six to seven days. After you complete three treatments with this mixture, use the yellow dock formula below to kill the mites.

HOW TO CLEAN YOUR CAT'S EARS

It's okay for your cat to have a small amount of wax in his ears, because this wax actually helps keep the ear tissues healthy. Any significant accumulation of debris, dirt, or wax, however, should be gently removed.

Gather up your supplies and have them within arm's reach (or have a family member help you). You want to make the ear cleaning experience as stress-free as possible for your cat (and you!)

You will need either a few drops of warm oil (see "Oil and Vitamin E" under "Home Remedies" above), diluted vinegar (three drops of white vinegar mixed in 1 ounce of water), or a commercial ear cleaning solution for cats, plus several cotton balls and/or a soft cotton cloth.

Hold the cat on your lap facing away from you.

Using an ear or eye dropper, place a few drops of your chosen ear cleaner into your cat's ear canal. Do not go deep with the dropper: The liquid will enter the canal by itself.

Massage the base of the ear with your thumb and forefinger. This loosens the wax and dirt. Some cats enjoy the massage.

Allow your cat to shake her head, then gently wipe out the ear with a cotton ball or a soft cloth.

Repeat on the other ear.

Yellow Dock

After you have cleaned your cat's ears using either the oil and vitamin E formula or another choice, the next step is treatment with yellow dock (*Rumex crispus*), which can kill those tiny pests. Treatment is simple: Combine 3 drops of yellow dock tincture in 1 tablespoon of filtered or distilled water. Use a dropper filled halfway to place the mixture in your cat's ear canal and massage the ear gently, starting at the base so the remedy gets into the ear. Allow your kitty to shake his head, then use a soft cotton cloth to blot away any excess liquid. Repeat this treatment once every three days for up to three weeks.

Yellow dock can also be used during the third step of mite treatment when you treat the entire cat with a bath. After you shampoo your cat, use a cooled yellow dock tea as the final rinse. To prepare the tea, add one heaping teaspoon of dried yellow dock to one cup of boiling water. Allow the herb to steep for 15 to 20 minutes in a covered pot or container. Cool before use.

Calendula

Calendula, better known as pot marigold (*Calendula offici-nalis*), has a long history as a popular herbal remedy for various skin conditions ranging from wounds to inflammation, rashes, and infections. Calendula flowers contain a variety of potentially helpful substances, including volatile oil, carotenoids, plant resin, and an assortment of other phytochemicals (plant chemicals). Although a preparation of calendula tea (cooled) won't kill ear mites, it can help reduce skin irritation and make your kitty feel better. To make a calendula remedy, combine ½ teaspoon of calendula tincture with ¼ teaspoon sea salt and ½ cup warm filtered water. Use a dropper or ear syringe to squeeze about ½ dropper of the mixture into your cat's ear. Massage the base of the ear and allow the mixture to be distributed in the ear canal. Then let your cat shake his head, after which you can wipe away any excess liquid with a soft cotton cloth. Treat the other ear.

Natural Mite Shampoos

Commercial shampoos designed to kill mites often contain ingredients that can irritate your cat's skin, such as parabens, sodium lauryl sulphate, and other chemicals. In fact, the directions on the shampoos tell you not to leave them on your cat for more than five to ten minutes specifically because they can cause skin problems.

You can, however, make your own mite shampoo that will eliminate the eggs, larvae, and adults. You will need to bathe your cat for three to four days in a row to get rid of the mites, but this shampoo will be kind to your cat's skin. The mite-elimination shampoo recipe is followed by another natural shampoo that will not get rid of mites, but it will soothe your cat's skin if he has been scratching himself.

For the mite-elimination shampoo, combine 200 ml (7 oz) of 1 or 2 percent hydrogen peroxide, 200 ml of warm water, 100 ml (3.5 oz) of borax and one 400 mg capsule of vitamin

E oil. Allow the borax to dissolve completely before you use the shampoo to bathe your cat. Work the shampoo into your cat's fur and skin. Rinse with plain water or, better yet, use a yellow dock rinse.

A shampoo that will soothe your cat's skin can be made using 200 ml (7 oz) of oatmeal ground in a food processor or coffee grinder, added to 1 cup of hot water. Allow the mixture to cool before using it to bathe your cat. Rinse your cat thoroughly with plain water or the yellow dock rinse.

Chapter 10
Feline Herpesvirus

A-choo! Does your kitty act like he has a cold? It could be feline herpesvirus, also known as feline viral rhinotracheitis, which is sometimes likened to the common cold in humans because the symptoms are similar. Feline herpesvirus is an acute upper respiratory condition caused by the feline herpesvirus type 1 (FHV-1). The virus attacks and infects the nose, throat, mouth, tonsils, sinus cavities, and eyes of a cat and causes a variety of symptoms characteristic of the common cold. Unlike the common cold, however, if you have a cat who has contracted FHV-1, he has it for life, even though this does not mean your cat will suffer symptoms all the time. In fact, many cats are latent carriers, which means they carry the virus but do not experience the symptoms or have only mild symptoms on occasion.

Feline herpesvirus is the most common cause of upper respiratory disease in cats. It's been estimated that 70 to 90 percent of cats are chronically infected with FHV-1. The first episode of FHV-1 in cats is typically the most severe, but once otherwise healthy cats recover from that outbreak, they usually manage to keep subsequent outbreaks to a minimum. The virus is capable of living in the body for a very long time, lying in wait until something triggers an attack.

Let's take a closer look at FHV-1 and what it means to cats who contract it.

WHO GETS FELINE HERPESVIRUS?

Cats most at risk for FHV-1 are kittens (especially those born to infected mothers) and older felines whose immune systems may not be as resilient as those of younger adult cats. Other cats at risk are those who live in multi-cat environments, such as a home with more than one cat, catteries, pet adoption centers and shelters, and pet stores. These cats typically share litter boxes as well as food and water bowls and toys. Both kittens and older cats also are at increased risk of dying of FHV-1.

A small number of cats seem to be more severely affected by FHV-1 virus than others, and it may be because they are experiencing several infections at the same time as their immune systems are compromised.

Cats who experience overcrowded conditions and stressful environments, who are in poor sanitary conditions, and who have poor nutrition are at greatest risk of the disease. Pregnant cats who are lactating and cats who have other health problems also are at high risk.

DOES MY CAT HAVE FELINE HERPESVIRUS?

Since FHV-1 is the most likely cause of upper respiratory disease, the telltale signs of feline herpes include many respiratory symptoms, such as sudden onset of sneezing, runny nose, discharge from the eyes, fever, eye ulcers, drooling, and loss of appetite, as well as conjunctivitis (see chapter 6), depression, ulcers in the mouth and on the tongue, and pneumonia. The symptoms typically last for about one week. If the affected cat is pregnant, spontaneous abortion may occur.

After a cat shows signs of feline herpesvirus and they subside and resolve, many cats develop secondary bacterial or other infections that can last for weeks or months. FHV-1 infection can become latent, meaning it goes into hiding and can reappear at any time in the future, although the symptoms tend to be less severe in these subsequent episodes.

Your cat could have FHV-1 and you may not know it because he doesn't display any symptoms. There are two possibilities. Asymptomatic carrier cats may shed the virus and infect other cats even though they don't have any symptoms. The virus is transmitted by oral and respiratory secretions either by direct contact (e.g., cats who groom each other or who get into a fight) or indirect contact, as when an infected cat who is shedding infects food bowls or bedding. Other cats with FHV-1 may be in a latent phase, during which they have no symptoms and do not shed the virus. A pregnant cat can pass the virus to her unborn kittens. Pregnant cats who catch herpes also may experience a spontaneous abortion.

DIAGNOSING FELINE HERPESVIRUS

Your veterinarian will conduct a physical examination and ask you whether your cat has been around other cats, when the symptoms started, what types of stress may have triggered the outbreak, and similar questions. Typically veterinarians take a swab from the mucous membranes and have it evaluated for polymerase chain reaction (PCR), which can significantly magnify the herpes virus. The PCR is not foolproof, however, and a cat can have FHV-1 even though the test comes back negative.

Several other diseases have symptoms that are similar to those of feline herpesvirus, so your veterinarian will want to rule these out. One of those diseases is calicivirus, which, like FHV-1, also can cause upper respiratory infections in cats. However, one distinguishing characteristic between these two viral conditions is that calicivirus usually causes ulcers in the mouth, whereas FHV-1 causes ulcers in the eye.

In fact, feline herpesvirus-1 is the most common cause of corneal ulcers in cats. If your cat has a corneal ulcer, your veterinarian will likely assume your cat has FHV-1 unless a different diagnosis can be proven. However, the presence of corneal ulcers is an important clue to FHV-1 and also a warning to begin antiviral treatment immediately to help prevent damage to the eye.

PREVENTING FELINE HERPESVIRUS

Most cats are exposed to calicivirus and/or herpesvirus type I at some time during their lives, and once exposed, the viruses stay for life. However, you may prevent any outbreaks of infectious upper respiratory tract infections or at least minimize their severity in your cat if she is vaccinated with the feline calicivirus/herpesvirus type I vaccine and its boosters. In most cases, healthy vaccinated cats keep the virus or viruses in check, and unless they experience a great deal of stress (e.g., pregnancy, boarding), they will probably not have an outbreak. Vaccination is recommended for all cats.

CONVENTIONAL TREATMENT

The goal of treatment for cats who have FHV-1 infection is to stop the virus from spreading, resolve secondary bacterial infections, relieve any pain, and minimize recurrence of the disease. Any cat who is showing signs of an upper respiratory infection should be checked by a veterinarian to determine if he has a fever, is dehydrated, or needs medication. Cats who are sneezing but not showing any other symptoms and who are acting normally probably don't need any treatment. However, if your cat shows any other signs, such as a runny nose, this is evidence of an infection.

The good news is that many cats who experience FHV-1 require little treatment other than some medication or home remedies (see "Home Remedies" below). Veterinarians typically prescribe an oral antibiotic or antiviral medication to fight the infection and relieve symptoms, while eyedrops or topical creams (e.g., atropine ointment) may be prescribed for conjunctivitis or other eye problems such as corneal ulcers (see chapter 6, "Conjunctivitis").

Idoxuridine is one of the more common antiviral medications veterinarians will prescribe for eye problems associated with FHV-1. This topical medication needs to be applied three to five times a day for several weeks until the corneal ulcer, conjunctivitis, or other eye infection clears, and then treatment should continue daily for an additional week to help ensure the infection does not return. This treatment program can be a challenge for pet parents, especially if they are not home during the day to administer the frequent doses. And need I mention how much cats enjoy having medication put into their eyes?

At the other end of the scale are cats who may need intravenous fluids and nutritional support via IV feedings. Fortunately, most cats do not advance to this stage. In reality, most cats who get feline herpesvirus have a successful recovery if they receive treatment, a nutritious diet, and loving care, even though they will likely have more episodes in the future.

One critical step is to separate the infected cat from any other cats and pets in the house because the condition is so contagious. Once one cat has FHV-1, any other cats in the house should be vaccinated if they have not been already.

HOME REMEDIES

Home remedies can be instrumental in caring for a cat who has feline herpesvirus. These home remedies can provide an added level of stability, comfort, and health to your cat's life. Let's look at how to provide loving home care to your cat with feline herpesvirus.

Diet

Kitties who contract FHV-1 often lose their sense of smell, which means they also often lose interest in food. Therefore, it's important to encourage your cat to eat nutritious food while he is experiencing a bout of FHV-1. Foods that have a strong odor, such as fish or food to which fish oil has been added, can be an incentive for cats to eat. You can try feeding high-quality canned food or a homemade recipe and adding a small amount of tuna water (from tuna packed in water, not oil) to entice your picky eater.

Colloidal Silver

Colloidal silver is a suspension of silver in a liquid solution, usually water, that is mainly used as an antiseptic. Although there is some controversy over the risks and benefits of colloidal silver, many states still require that newborns be administered eyedrops of silver nitrate to prevent eye infections, so it is still considered valuable for some aspects of health. In cats who have feline herpesvirus, colloidal silver may be useful in two ways. One way is to use undiluted colloidal silver (in a concentration of less than 50 parts per million [ppm], preferably 30 ppm) in a warm eye compress to wipe your cat's eyes to remove any discharge.

Colloidal silver also can be used internally to fight the virus: ½ teaspoon two to three times per day for one week, followed by ½ teaspoon every two to three days for one week, then stop treatment. Use a colloidal silver product that is 10 ppm or 30 ppm. A rare side effect associated with using colloidal silver is called argyria, in which the skin turns gray/silver because the body has accumulated an excessive amount of silver. This typically is not a concern with cats, so you shouldn't see your white short-haired transform into a silver-gray feline!

Elderberry

The herb elderberry (*Sambucus nigra* L.) is a shrubby tree that has white flowers that are rich in vitamins A, B, and C and other substances that can help fight viruses. Elderberry tea is known for its ability to help fight colds in people, and cats can benefit from this herb as well. To make elderberry tea, steep 3 to 5 grams of dried elderberry flowers in 8 ounces of boiling water for ten to fifteen minutes. After the tea has cooled, give a dropperful of the tea to your cat two to three times a day. If your kitty will not cooperate, then try giving her ⅛ teaspoon of a nonalcohol elderberry extract on her food.

Lysine

Lysine is an essential amino acid that has an ability to suppress replication of the FHV-1 virus. Supplementation with lysine can be effective in relieving symptoms of FHV-1. You can expect the best results if you start supplementation as soon as symptoms begin. A typical starting dose is 500 mg per day for up to one week, which is then reduced to 250 mg as a maintenance dose for a week or two. Because lysine competes with another amino acid (arginine), do not continue with the 250-mg maintenance dose for a prolonged time. Cats who get feline herpes can experience flare-ups of the disease anytime throughout their lives, and lysine is a suggested supplement to give to your cat when symptoms return.

Vaporizer

Cats with FHV-1 can benefit greatly from having a vaporizer or humidifier in the area they occupy the most. The addition of several drops of eucalyptus or peppermint oil to the reservoir in the vaporizer can help relieve any breathing problems. Keep your sick kitty in a room by himself at night or for several hours per day with the vaporizer until symptoms clear.

Stress Reduction

It's often difficult to know what will "stress out" your cat. Do you have a new baby? Did you forgot to clean the litter box? Did you move the recliner from the left side of the room to the right? Is your cat alone all day?

Naturally, every cat responds to situations in a different way, but after a while pet parents can usually identify which general types of circumstances or actions will cause stress in their cat. The main trigger for recurring episodes of infection is stress. Once you are aware of potential stressors and how to alleviate their impact, you can take small steps to make your cat's life—and yours as well—more stress-free and comfortable.

With that said, here are some possible stress reducers.

- ✓ **Be sure your cat has things to do to distract her.** Toys that require her to interact, such as a circular tube with a ball in it she can hit, hanging feathers or other objects, or a toy she can swat are possibilities, especially ones that are filled with dry catnip. Cats enjoy watching the world go by, so if there is at least one window she can look out of, be sure she has room to sit and watch; you may need to supply a window seat. For some cats, a good distraction is another cat: if you are not already a two-cat home, you might consider adopting a shelter cat. Two cats can keep each other company, groom each other, and perhaps play together.

- ✓ **Provide human contact.** It's critical that you or other family members spend time with your cat every day playing, grooming, or just hanging out and stroking. If you are away all day, do you have a neighbor who might drop by occasionally and spend time with your cat? Elderly individuals or people who are home a lot might like to spend some quality time with your kitty.

- ✓ **Offer heights.** Cats enjoy climbing on top of things, such as cupboards, refrigerators, and even curtain rods (unfortunately). Being high makes them feel safe. Provide your cat with something safe to climb, such as a cat tree.

- ✓ **Hire a cat sitter.** If you and your family need to go away, consider hiring a cat sitter rather than putting your cat in a kennel or boarding facility. The fact you are leaving the cat is stressful enough, but "abandoning her" (that's how a cat may view it) in a strange

environment is even worse. If you have someone
either stay with the cat or visit once or twice a day
for feeding and play time while you are gone, this
can significantly reduce the stress related with your
departure.

✓ **Reduce impact of a new family member.** Did you
just add a new baby to your family? Did your son
or daughter come back home to live? Has your
mother-in-law moved in? These new people in the
house can cause stress for your cat, especially if the
person is a stranger. Be sure to offer your cat places
where she will feel safe: a cat tree, a room of her
own, a corner with several boxes she can hide in.

✓ **Keep the litter box clean.** Every cat has his own
level of tolerance when it comes to a litter box.
Some cats will put up with a box that isn't cleaned
out after every use, while others act out if the box
is not always clean. If your cat is of the latter sort,
provide two litter boxes so you can stay ahead of
the game.

At Ohio State University, a three-year study examined
the impact of stress on cat health. (It was even funded by the
National Institutes of Health!) Twelve healthy cats and twenty
cats with feline interstitial cystitis (a painful urinary tract
condition) were involved in the study. During the first part
of the study, the researchers interacted with the cats in a con-
sistent manner by cleaning their cages and litter boxes, providing food and toys, playing music, and spending time with
them.

When the cats were exposed to moderate stressors (e.g., a
loud noise, a dirty litter box), they responded by urinating or
defecating outside the litter box, eating less, or vomiting. In
fact, when stressors were introduced to the cats, they got sick
twice as much as they did when they were not exposed to
stress. When the stressors were stopped, the cats returned to
their normal state, which was getting sick or acting out about
once per week.

The take-home message is that stress can cause illness in cats, just as it can in people. It's important to recognize stressors and take steps to minimize them for your cat, especially when he has feline herpesvirus.

HELPFUL AT-HOME TIPS TO RELIEVE FHV-1 SYMPTOMS

✓ Help clear your cat's eyes, nose, and mouth with cotton balls soaked in warm water or in herbal remedies (see "Home Remedies").

✓ If your cat is reluctant to eat, try a combination of the following foods: 1 teaspoon each of pureed raw liver, chicken baby food, cottage cheese, and fish oil. This food combination is generally tempting to most cats.

✓ Give the following vitamin supplements, which can support your cat's health: 100 IU vitamin E twice per week; 250 mg vitamin C twice daily for 14 days; and ¼ vitamin B complex once daily.

✓ Use a vaporizer as recommended above.

Chapter 11

Fleas

I wish someone could tell me one good reason why we need fleas, because I know there are millions of pet parents out there, like myself, who would love to see them disappear. And so would our cats.

Cat fleas are a significant problem in many parts of the United States, and especially the *Ctenocephalides felis*, or cat flea. These pesky critters thrive in humidity, which is why cat flea problems are more prominent in the Deep South, Middle Atlantic states, the Gulf Coast, and parts of the Midwest than they are in Colorado, Arizona, or California.

When fleas take up shelter in your cat, they bite and inject their saliva, which causes allergic reactions, called flea allergy dermatitis, in many cats. Fleas also can carry and transmit a variety of infectious agents, including the larvae of the tapeworm. Cats can become infested with the worms if they ingest fleas while grooming. Because fleas feed on blood, they can cause anemia in vulnerable kittens. And let's not forget that when your cat has fleas, so does your house!

DOES MY CAT HAVE FLEAS?

Cats can scratch for several reasons, so if your cat is having a scratchfest, it doesn't necessarily mean fleas have moved in. However, there are several ways to tell if your cat has fleas. One, run your hand through her coat and part the fur. Fleas generally like to populate areas around the ears, belly, and armpits. Look for live fleas and be prepared for some fast-moving pests. Although fleas can't fly, they have six legs and can jump as high and far as four feet, so you may see some activity while you are searching. You also may see flea dirt, which is flea feces that looks like tiny black specks. When you rub these specks, they will leave a red-brown stain.

If you have a long-haired cat or your cat does not cooperate with a close inspection, another way to look for fleas is to place your cat on a white sheet of paper and comb her with a flea comb or brush. You should see fleas and/or flea dirt on the white sheet. If you have more than one cat and you think only one cat has fleas, think again. Fleas are very opportunistic and will infest all your cats, and dogs too. (Yes, dogs get the same fleas that cats get.)

HOW TO TREAT MORE THAN YOUR CAT FOR FLEAS

If your cat has fleas, your house does as well, and you may be experiencing some flea bites too. Unfortunately, just treating your cat is not enough to guarantee the fleas will be gone: If flea eggs, larvae, or adults are in your furniture, rugs, or other places in your house, they can keep on infesting your cat. It's been said that for every flea you see on your cat, there are about one hundred more in your house. Here are some nontoxic home remedies for ridding your home of fleas:

- ✓ Vacuum your home thoroughly, including the furniture, rugs, and anything covered in fabric. Throw out the vacuum bag.
- ✓ Keep carpets, throw rugs, and anything made of fabric as dry as possible. Moisture and humidity promote fleas.
- ✓ Steam clean your carpets and floors to remove flea larvae.
- ✓ Wash throw rugs and bedding.

(*continued*)

✓ Treat carpeting with diatomaceous earth (food-grade; see "Home Remedies" on page 136) or a boric acid-based powder. Sprinkle the product on your carpet, brush it in using a broom, then vacuum. Both diatomaceous earth and boric acid powders are effective against flea larvae but will not harm pets or people, including children.

✓ Capture fleas using a homemade trap. Hang a light source over a piece of flypaper or a bowl of soapy water, and the light will attract the fleas to the paper or water.

✓ Treat your yard and garden. If your cat goes outdoors, or if you have a dog that goes outdoors, you may need to treat your yard as well. This may seem like a daunting task, but concentrate on spots where fleas like to breed, such as shady, moist areas. Clean up any wet leaves, pine needles, and debris from under trees, bushes, and decks. A safe, natural way to treat the yard is with microscopic worms called nematodes, which feast on flea larvae and grubs but don't harm your lawn garden, pets, or family. Diatomaceous earth also can be used in your yard. Both of these products should be available at a garden center.

CONVENTIONAL TREATMENT

If you are going to choose a conventional treatment for your cat's fleas, one of the most important things you should remember is to *never* use a dog flea product on your cat. Cats are much more sensitive to some products and ingredients than are dogs. In addition, kittens and adult cats typically must use different products or at least different doses of a product, so be sure you read the instructions carefully.

There are a wide variety of products both over-the-counter and by prescription, ranging from flea collars to sprays, shampoos, topical medications, and pills. Flea collars are largely believed to be ineffective and may even cause skin irritation. Shampoos can be helpful, but simple home-remedy shampoos can be just as effective as more costly and possibly irritating commercial brands. (See "Home Remedies" on page 136.) Many veterinarians prefer monthly flea-preventive programs that are applied to the back of the cat's neck or given by mouth and contain substances that can interfere with the life cycle of the fleas. Here is a representative list of some of these products so you can get an idea of their ingredients, uses, and side effects. Generally, none of these products should be used by cats who are elderly, ill, pregnant, or younger than eight weeks of age unless otherwise noted on the package.

- **Advantage II.** This topical medication kills fleas at all stages of the life cycle. Advantage II contains the insecticide imidacloprid and the insect growth regulator pyriproxyfen. Imidacloprid is not absorbed into the bloodstream or tissues well, so toxicity is usually not a problem. Cats who lick it (imidacloprid is very bitter) will drool profusely. Some cats may experience hair loss at the application site.
- **Bio Spot Spot On.** This topical product kills adult fleas using the insecticide fipronil. Fipronil is not absorbed by your cat's body, but it is stored in the oil glands of the skin. Some cats experienced irritation at the application site, as well as rash or swelling.
- **Frontline Top Spot.** This also contains fipronil (see above warning).
- **Frontline Plus.** Contains fipronil plus S-methoprene, an insect growth regulator, which can eliminate fleas at all stages of life.
- **Revolution.** The main ingredient in this product is selamectin, which kills not only fleas but ear mites and some ticks. Because this product accumulates in

skin oils and hair follicles and lingers in the bloodstream, it can cause allergic reactions in some cats.
Hair loss at the application site can occur, while
rare side effects may include vomiting, diarrhea,
drooling, muscle tremors, and loss of appetite.

HOME REMEDIES

A cat who eats a high-quality, natural diet and whose immune system is strong is less likely to experience problems
with fleas, or at least be much less bothered by them. Therefore, your first line of defense against fleas is a healthy
diet, as discussed in the early chapters. Once your cat has
fleas, however, it's time to call in a line of home remedy
strategies, and they can include the suggestions below.

Use your own judgment, however. If your cat is heavily
infested with fleas, he will likely need a conventional treatment approach, but then follow up with home remedies. For
cats who have mild or moderate problems with fleas, home
remedies may be all they need. Because natural approaches
don't have the staying power (or the toxicity) of chemical
treatments, you typically need to use them more often or for
a longer period of time.

Apple Cider Vinegar

While apple cider vinegar won't kill fleas, applying it to your
cat's coat and skin will help if she has flea bite dermatitis. If
your cat is suffering with flea bites, try this trick. Combine
equal parts apple cider vinegar and water, 2 ounces of each.
Place it in a spray bottle and spritz your cat's fur, working the
liquid down to the skin. Be careful not to spray your cat's face.

Brewer's Yeast

A teaspoon of brewer's yeast in your cat's food each day
may chase the fleas away. Why? Because apparently fleas

are not fond of thiamine, and brewer's yeast is especially rich in this B vitamin. When your cat eats the yeast, it can be detected through the skin by fleas and they leave. You will need to give the yeast to your cat daily for at least four weeks before it will be effective. Therefore, brewer's yeast can be a good preventive if you start dosing your cat before flea season begins. Some cats are allergic to this yeast, so if your cat begins to scratch or shows signs of a skin allergy, stop the dosage.

Another option is to sprinkle brewer's yeast on your cat's fur and rub it in. This approach should give you faster results.

Citrus

The main component of citrus peel oil, D-limonene, can destroy fleas at all stages of their life. Some flea products contain this citrus extract, but you can prepare your own. Place 16 ounces of water in a saucepan and bring it to a rapid boil. Slice a large unpeeled lemon into the water, cover, and remove from the heat. Allow the lemon to steep overnight. Strain the liquid through cheesecloth. Be sure the liquid is at room temperature or cooler before you put it into a spray bottle. Spritz your cat, thoroughly rubbing the citrus water into the fur and skin, avoiding his eyes and genital area. Treat your cat once a day or as needed.

Diatomaceous Earth

Diatomaceous earth is a safe, nontoxic substance made from the finely ground skeletons of diatoms, which are one-celled plants that live in the water. Their fossiled remains are gathered in chalky deposits called diatomite, which is composed primarily of silicon (33 percent), calcium (19 percent), and lesser amounts of iron, magnesium, sodium, and trace minerals. Diatomaceous earth is available as a white powder in several grades, including food-grade and garden/pool-grade. Be sure you buy food-grade diatomaceous earth to treat your cat, as the other product can harm your kitty.

Sprinkle 1 tablespoon of diatomaceous earth along your cat's spine and rub it into the fur against the way the hair is growing. There's no need to rub it hard into the skin, however. Use another tablespoon to treat the rest of her body, especially the belly, armpits, legs, and paws. Diatomaceous earth may look harmless, but if you look at it under a microscope, you will see it is made up of particles that have razor-sharp edges. But not to worry: The minute daggers harm only fleas, not your cat. Once the particles pierce the fleas, they die of dehydration. One precaution with diatomaceous earth: Apply it gently and try not to breathe in the dust because it can irritate some people and cats. After the dust has settled, there is no problem.

If your cat has many fleas, you may want to bathe him first, use a flea comb to get fleas that have been left behind, and then allow your cat to thoroughly dry before applying diatomaceous earth. For heavy flea problems, use diatomaceous earth daily until the fleas subside, then once every three to four days until they disappear completely. (Remember, however, to treat your house as well.)

Rosemary

Rosemary (*Rosmarinus officinalis*) is an aromatic herb that can help repel fleas. If you don't already have a rosemary bush in your yard, get one, because you'll find that it can help year-round. One way to discourage fleas is to grind fresh rosemary leaves and sprinkle them where your cat likes to sleep. You can also steep ¼ cup of fresh rosemary leaves in 8 ounces of boiling water for thirty minutes, then strain out the herb. Dilute the rosemary tea with ½ gallon of warm water and use it to bathe your cat, or give her a spritz bath and rub the diluted tea into her fur. Rosemary also has anti-inflammatory properties, so if your cat has skin irritation because of flea bites, the rosemary can help relieve itching.

Shampoo

There's nothing fancy about these flea shampoos: simple, mild dishwashing detergent, gentle castile soap, or black soap. If you're up for giving your cat a bath, add several drops of a mild dishwashing detergent or liquid castile soap to the bathwater or lather up some black soap and work it into your cat's fur and watch the fleas die. Be sure to rinse your cat well, however, because even mild soap may cause skin reactions in some cats. After you rinse off the soapy water, you might try a final rinse with yellow dock (see page 119) to soothe his skin.

Chapter 12

Hair Balls

It's wonderful how cats try to keep themselves well groomed and clean, but a side effect of their fastidiousness is hair balls. What pet parent hasn't come across a wet hair ball in the center of the carpet or, worse, stepped on one with bare feet in the middle of the night?

You cat cannot digest the hair she licks and swallows, but much of it passes through her stomach and intestinal tract with nary a problem. Sometimes, however, especially during times of heavy shedding and among long-haired cats, the hair accumulates in the stomach and forms a hair ball, known in scientific circles as a trichobezoar.

How can you deal with this common but annoying and occasionally disgusting problem? Here's a quick look at everything you ever wanted to know (or perhaps didn't) about hair balls and how to deal with them.

TELL ME ABOUT HAIR BALLS

There's no need to have a heading called "Does My Cat Have Hair Balls?" because you've likely already identified the icky proof in the middle of the rug or kitchen floor. However, what you may not know is something about the hair balls themselves and your cat's ability to deal with them.

The fact is cats have a digestive system designed to handle hair, its own as well as that of any prey it manages to catch and consume. Just because your cat may not include mice and other furry critters as part of its diet does not mean its digestive tract can't handle its own fur. However, today's domestic cats have fur that is often longer than that of its ancestors, so it's believed this is one reason why today's house cats can't manage to pass all of the accumulated hair out of their intestinal tracts. That means the hair ball comes back via the same route by which it entered the stomach.

If your cat vomits a hair ball once a month or even every few weeks and she isn't displaying any symptoms, such as loss of appetite or bowel problems, then chances are your cat is handling any hair she is ingesting just fine. However, if your cat is passing hair balls several times a week or every day, or if she is having difficulty bringing up a hair ball (it should come up after one or two tries), then it's time to see your veterinarian.

DIAGNOSING HAIR BALLS

Although it may seem rather obvious when a cat coughs up hair balls, these squishy "gifts" from your cat can be serious if they occur often. In some cats, hair balls can block the throat, intestinal tract, or stomach. Cats who are having difficulty with hair balls may experience other symptoms, such as diarrhea, problems with defecation (straining but nothing comes out), loss of appetite, a bloated abdomen, and lethargy. It's time to see your veterinarian if your cat is coughing and producing a hacking sound and no hair ball emerges from her throat. Hacking without expelling a hair ball can be a sign of asthma, so it's a good idea to have your cat checked by a veterinarian if she displays these symptoms or if she is often coughing up hair balls.

Other signs of a hair ball that could be a serious problem are vomiting, lack of appetite, constipation, lethargy, and diarrhea. Your veterinarian will ask you about these and any other symptoms your cat may be experiencing.

CONVENTIONAL TREATMENT

Various hairball remedies are on the market, and they tend to consist of mineral oil or petroleum jelly along with something tasty, such as malt or tuna flavor, so your cat will eat it. These pastes lubricate the digestive tract, allowing hairballs to pass easily through the intestines and exit with the feces. You can easily make your own lubricant at home and save money (see "Home Remedies" below).

Cat food makers also produce cat food specifically for management of hair balls. These foods usually have up to ten times the amount of fiber normally found in cat food, along with added digestive enzymes. Since cats need only a very limited amount of carbohydrates and fiber, these diets can not only irritate the gastrointestinal tract, but also cause either loose or hard stools as well as an increase in the number of feces and an increased need for water intake. They also may cause your cat to produce more concentrated urine, which makes your kitty more susceptible to a urinary tract infection. Yet another problem with high-fiber foods for hairballs is they may not help eliminate hairballs that get stuck in the stomach. Overall, these foods are not healthy for your cat, and home remedies can be a better choice.

HOME REMEDIES

The home remedy approach to hair balls involves both prevention and treatment. With regular attention, hairballs can be a thing of the past, or at least not present a problem for your cat.

Diet

Pet parents who prepare homemade food for their cats generally report less of a hair ball problem with their cats. Rather than rely on special commercial hair ball cat foods,

the addition of a *small* amount of fiber to your cat's diet—
such as in the form of pumpkin (see "Pumpkin" on page
144) or ⅛ of a teaspoon of ground psyllium (see "Slippery
Elm" on page 144) or flaxseed to her food every two to three
days—can be adequate for cats who have occasional difficulty with hair balls. Otherwise, cats who are groomed regularly and who eat a homemade or high-quality wet commercial
diet rarely have any unusual problems with hair balls.

Grooming

Probably the best home remedy is to attempt to prevent hair
balls from happening at all, and as a pet parent you can
facilitate that effort by grooming your cat regularly. Yes,
your kitty is probably doing a great job all by herself, but
she is also gathering up the ingredients for a hair ball during
the process. Use a fine-tooth comb on short-haired cats, but
long-haired varieties need a wider-tooth comb, preferably
one that has revolving teeth.

Daily combing may be best during the summer months,
when cats seem to shed the most, while twice or three times
a week may be adequate other times during the year. How
much grooming you should do really depends on your cat.
If your cat absolutely hates to be groomed, you may need to
occasionally take her to a professional.

Lubricant

For decades, the home remedy for hair balls has been petroleum jelly, and it still works. The reason for its success is
that the intestines cannot absorb the molecules, so the jelly
passes out of the cat's intestinal tract unchanged, bringing
the hair along with it. If your cat is experiencing hair balls,
give him about ⅛ of a teaspoon on your finger and let him
lick it off. Try giving your cat petroleum jelly for three to
four days, then switch to once a week as a way to prevent
hair balls. For fussy cats, you can place the glob of lubricant
on your cat's leg just under the elbow (if you put it on a paw,

he's likely to flick it off). Granted, petroleum jelly isn't the most tasty treat, so you might want to jazz it up with tuna water (from tuna packed in water) or even a tiny amount of ground chicken.

You might also try a small amount of mineral oil, which can be equally challenging to get cats to consume. Mineral oil is the main ingredient in most commercially available hair ball products, and it has a more laxative effect than does petroleum jelly, so beware! If you are thinking about substituting other slippery type substances, such as fish oil or olive oil, to do the job, they are absorbed by the intestinal tract and won't provide the effect you want.

Pumpkin

Plain canned pumpkin (without any added flavorings) can help improve the elimination of hair balls. Many cats enjoy the taste of canned pumpkin, which provides a reasonable amount of fiber, while other cats do not like it. One tablespoon of canned pumpkin twice daily can help send those nasty hair balls on their way. Try the pumpkin for two to three days and then see how your kitty responds. If the hairballs should return, give her pumpkin for another few days.

Slippery Elm

A study published in the *Journal of Nutrition* reported that a chew product containing both slippery elm and psyllium husks helped cats who had chronic problems with hair balls. The researchers tested the product against a placebo in twenty-four cats. The study was a randomized, placebo-controlled crossover design, which means half the cats were randomly assigned to receive the product for two weeks, while the other half were given the placebo. Then the groups were switched: Cats who had originally tried the hair ball product were given the placebo, and those who had had the placebo were given the product for two weeks.

When the cats enjoyed the slippery elm and psyllium product, the pet parents reported 29 percent fewer signs of hair balls (coughing, retching, vomiting) than when the cats got placebo. This suggests that slippery elm, as well as psyllium, may be helpful in managing hair balls in cats.

Chapter 13

Hyperthyroidism

Hyperthyroidism, or an overactive thyroid gland, is the most common hormone disorder that affects cats. This condition is characterized by the overproduction of the hormone thyroxine (T4), a substance that increases the rate of cell metabolism. Hyperthyroidism is most often seen in middle-aged and older cats, with the average age of onset being just younger than thirteen years. In fact, only 5 percent of cats with the disease develop the disease before they are eight years old.

Hyperthyroidism can affect cats of any sex or breed, although there is some suggestion that Siamese cats are less likely to develop the disorder. In any case, hyperthyroidism can have a significant impact on a cat's body and quality of life. Fortunately, hyperthyroidism is treatable in the majority of cases, and cats with the disorder can live long, happy lives with appropriate treatment.

WHAT IS THE THYROID GLAND?

The thyroid gland is an endocrine gland that produces hormones responsible for regulating a variety of metabolic processes and calcium balance in the body. The elongated gland consists of two lobes, one on each side of the windpipe, and is located in the front of the neck below the voice box. Two of the hormones produced by the gland, T3 and T4, stimulate tissues in the body to produce proteins and increase the amount of oxygen the cells use. A third hormone, calcitonin, works with the parathyroid hormone to regulate levels of calcium in the body.

The thyroid gland does not work alone: The amount of hormone secreted by the thyroid is controlled by the amount of thyroid-stimulating hormone produced by the pituitary gland. In turn, the production of thyroid-stimulating hormone is controlled by an area of the brain called the hypothalamus.

DOES MY CAT HAVE HYPERTHYROIDISM?

Your cat may have hyperthyroidism if she displays the following symptoms. The numbers indicate the percentage of cats with the disease who typically have the sign or symptom:

- Unexplained weight loss: 90 percent
- Excessive hunger/increased food consumption: 53 percent
- Vomiting: 44 percent
- Excessive water consumption/urination: 40 percent
- Hair loss and/or poor coat: 30 percent
- Diarrhea: 20 percent
- Tremor: 15 percent
- Weakness: 13 percent
- Panting or difficulty breathing: 12 percent
- Reduced level of activity: 12 percent
- Loss of appetite: 7 percent.

Hyperthyroidism has far-reaching effects and can impact many organs of the body, causing secondary problems. Cats with hyperthyroidism are often restless or hyperactive, and some become intolerant of heat. They may experience a rapid heart rate, heart murmurs, and high blood pressure. The good news is that if hyperthyroidism is treated, heart-related problems often improve and may disappear completely. If hyperthyroidism is not treated, cats may develop a heart condition called hypertrophic cardiomyopathy, which causes a cat's heart muscle to thicken and can result in heart failure and death.

Sometimes cats experience both hyperthyroidism and kidney disease (chronic kidney failure; see chapter 15), a relatively common condition in older cats. This combination of disorders can be tricky to treat, because hyperthyroidism can increase blood supply to the kidneys, which can hide a severe problem with kidney function. In such case, cats need to be monitored closely with regular blood and urine tests.

CAUSES OF HYPERTHYROIDISM

Hyperthyroidism is most often caused by a noncancerous (benign) accumulation or growth of cells (nodules) in the thyroid gland. These nodules, which are also called adenomas, make up about 70 percent of cases of hyperthyroidism in cats. Fortunately, only 1 to 2 percent of hyperthyroidism is associated with thyroid cancer. An iodine deficiency may also contribute to hyperthyroidism, and in fact a recent study suggested that cat food makers reevaluate the levels of iodine in cat food since many foods may be deficient.

Veterinarians have been seeing an increase in the number of cats with hyperthyroidism in the past several decades. Although the exact reasons for this increase is not known, experts speculate that diet and environmental and immunological factors may be involved. One theory is that canned food and not being purebred are risk factors for hyperthyroidism. Since dried food is viewed as an overall poor choice for nutrition because of its high carbohydrate levels, pet parents may be left with considering homemade food for their cats.

Another theory is that the rise in hyperthyroidism has parallelled the increase in the number of vaccinations cats are given, including those recommended yearly. Such vaccines challenge the immune system and attack the thyroid gland in some cats.

Yet here is one more possible contributing factor to the rise in hyperthyroidism in domestic cats, and the source may surprise you. A study was conducted by scientists at the Environmental Protection Agency (EPA), who looked at introduction of polybrominated diphenyl ethers (or PBDEs, flame retardant fabrics that can disrupt hormones) into items commonly found in the house (e.g., clothing, upholstered furniture, carpeting, drapes) and the parallel dramatic rise in hyperthyroidism in cats. Unfortunately, PBDEs are also found in canned foods, including cat foods. The authors discovered that canned cat food containing fish and/or seafood had higher PBDE levels than non-seafood canned foods.

Overall, the scientists found that cats with hyperthyroidism had much higher blood levels of PBDEs than cats without the disease. Since dry cat food is not recommended and canned foods may contain PBDEs, what's a pet parent to do? You can switch to homemade foods and/or place leftover canned cat food in a glass jar, especially those containing fish or seafood.

DIAGNOSING HYPERTHYROIDISM

Veterinarians rely on reports from pet parents concerning any symptoms of hyperthyroidism their cat may be experiencing. Your vet will also palpate (feel and lightly press) your cat's neck to feel for the thyroid gland. Although the thyroid gland of a healthy cat cannot be palpated, most cats with hyperthyroidism have an enlarged thyroid that can be detected easily. Infrequently, the thyroid grows so large it sinks into the chest cavity.

Diagnosis of hyperthyroidism also usually involves checking thyroid hormone levels. A high T4 level is a more reliable indicator of hyperthyroidism than is an elevated T3 level, because the latter is not elevated in about one-quarter of cats who have the disorder. Occasionally, cats with hyperthyroidism have a normal T4 level even though they have other clear signs of the disease. A repeat test usually reveals an elevated T4. Sometimes a veterinarian will also check the pancreas, because it produces thyroid stimulating hormone, which stimulates the thyroid to produce hormones.

Diseases such as diabetes, kidney failure, liver disease, and heart disease also display signs of hyperthyroidism, so your veterinarian may order laboratory tests, such as a complete blood count, serum chemistry, and urinalysis, to rule out or identify these conditions (especially kidney failure). However, it is also true that cats who develop hyperthyroidism frequently have one of these other conditions as well, which can make both diagnosis and treatment challenging.

Occasionally, a technetium scan (whereby a substance called technetium is injected into the cat and observed on the scan) may be suggested if surgery is being considered and the abnormal thyroid is not clearly identifiable using regular examination procedures. The results of these tests may also help your veterinarian decide which course of treatment is best for your cat.

CONVENTIONAL TREATMENT

If your cat has been diagnosed with hyperthyroidism, there are several conventional treatments available. Here is a brief explanation of the three main choices.

Drug Treatment

Two oral anti-thyroid drugs are available for cats: both work by reducing the production and release of thyroid hormone from the thyroid gland, and both need to be taken for the rest of a cat's life. Once a cat begins taking these medications, thyroid hormone concentrations usually reach a healthy range within three weeks, and then the dose can be adjusted. Both drugs are relatively inexpensive.

- **Methimazole** (Felimazole, Tapazole) is usually taken twice a day, although some cats need only one dose per day once they are stabilized. A transdermal form (gel) of methimazole has been developed for application on a cat's ear. Methimazole is also used presurgery in cats who are scheduled for removal of their thyroid (thyroidectomy).

- **Carbimazole** (Vidalta) is a slow-release formula, which means it can be taken once daily.

Both drugs are associated with mild side effects, including vomiting, lethargy, scratching of the face, and poor appetite, but these problems usually go away after the first few weeks of treatment and/or by temporarily reducing the dose and giving the medication with food. Infrequently, serious side effects such as a reduced white blood cell count, liver disorders, and skin irritation occur, and hypothyroidism (abnormally low production of thyroid hormone) occurs in rare cases.

Veterinarians often recommend medication as a first course of treatment because it can help reverse problems with metabolism and heart conditions associated with the disease. Use of medication also helps veterinarians better assess kidney function and kidney disease, which can occur along with hyperthyroidism.

Surgical Thyroidectomy

A potential long-term or permanent cure for hyperthyroidism is a thyroidectomy, or removal of the gland. Not every cat who has a thyroidectomy is cured, however, if not all the diseased tissue is removed or if previously unaffected thyroid tissue becomes affected at a later time. Potential danger associated with a thyroidectomy is accidental damage to the parathyroid glands, which lie close to the thyroid gland lobes. Damage to the parathyroid glands, which are responsible for regulating blood calcium levels, can result in a life-threatening drop in calcium concentrations in the bloodstream.

Radioactive Iodine Therapy

Radioactive iodine therapy is a safe, effective treatment for hyperthyroidism that usually results in a cure (95 percent of cases) with no further interventions required. Because this therapy requires handling a radioactive substance, only a limited number of facilities offer this treatment. Cats who undergo radioactive iodine therapy receive a single injection of the iodine, after which they need to stay hospitalized until their radiation level has reached a safe limit, which can take several weeks. Occasionally radioactive iodine therapy results in a permanent reduction in thyroid hormone levels, which means the cat must then be treated with thyroid hormone supplements.

HOME REMEDIES

Because hyperthyroidism involves the immune system, some veterinarians, especially those who practice holistic veterinary medicine, believe the first approach to treatment should involve modifications to the diet and nutrition. Therefore, those are the two approaches discussed here.

Diet

If your cat is not already eating a high-quality commercial diet or homemade food, an immediate switch is recommended. An all-natural diet can help reduce the overproduction of thyroid hormone and rebalance the immune system. Low-quality food, on the other hand, places excessive stress on the immune system and can cause the thyroid to overreact.

Some research has suggested that certain foods may contribute to the development of hyperthyroidism, so they should be avoided. These include soy (often found in canned cat food) as well as foods you might add to homemade cat food (although most are not usually recommended), such as sweet potatoes, lima beans, onions, garlic, millet, and cabbage. On the other hand, it's been shown that cats who regularly eat beef, chicken, or turkey have a reduced risk of hyperthyroidism.

I also mentioned earlier that canned foods, after they are opened, should be placed in a glass container because of possible PBDE contamination. This is especially important for canned foods that contain fish and/or seafood.

If you consider all of these caveats concerning diet and hyperthyroidism, you are still left with many dietary choices. Several recipes in chapter 1 are appropriate for cats who have hyperthyroidism, as is the following option:

Hyperthyroid Recipe

This provides six servings: three days of meals for a 10-lb cat.

1 lb ground beef or ground chicken
2 Tbs cooked mashed carrots or broccoli
4 tsp flaxseed, ground
2 Tbs cooked brown rice
½ cup water
2 multivitamin/mineral supplement (with taurine)
   for cats

Combine all the ingredients except the supplement in a saucepan and cook over low heat until the meat is done. Add more water if needed. When done, stir or pour in the supplement. If you are using a tablet, you will need to pulverize the supplement. You can double or triple this recipe and freeze the extra in a cupcake tin in ½ cup servings.

Coenzyme Q10

Coenzyme Q10 (CoQ10) is a substance that has antioxidant properties and is similar to a vitamin but has not been elevated to vitamin status. The body produces CoQ10 and uses it to manufacture energy for cell growth and maintenance. Every cell in the body contains some CoQ10, and it plays a significant role in protecting the body from damage.

Levels of CoQ10 tend to be low in people who have

hyperthyroidism as well as heart problems, and some holistic veterinarians suggest it may be helpful in cats as well. A
recommended daily dose is 30 to 50 mg to help relax excessive thyroid activity and thus reduce symptoms.

L-carnitine

L-carnitine is an amino acid produced by the body that is
involved in the metabolism of fat. Like coenzyme Q10,
L-carnitine may help calm the thyroid and thus provide relief from symptoms. A few studies in people offer evidence
that this supplement may be beneficial. One reported that
L-carnitine appeared to be helpful in both human and animal cells and that "carnitine would be useful both for the
prevention and the therapy of the thyroid storm." Thyroid
storm is a condition in which thyroid hormone levels rise
dramatically and symptoms become severe, especially body
temperature. Although thyroid storm is not common, it is
life threatening.

Chapter 14

Intestinal Worms

If you have an adult indoor cat, you may be thinking, *Worms? They only affect kittens and outdoor cats, right? I don't have to worry about worms, do I?* Unfortunately, both outdoor and indoor cats can and do get worms. In fact, these intestinal parasites can affect cats of any breed, age, size, or location. But there are steps you can take to remedy the situation.

One reason intestinal worms are a problem among domesticated cats is the fact that our feline companions *are* domesticated. A significant problem with domestication of cats is the commercial pet foods people have forced upon their cats. The further away cats are taken from the natural balance of macronutrients they need to thrive—high protein, moderately high fat, and minimal carbohydrates—the more difficult it is for their immune systems to keep the body in balance and to ward off infection and parasites, such as intestinal worms. Therefore the most basic and important thing you can do as a pet parent to avoid intestinal worms is to feed your cat food that promotes the goal of a balanced, healthy immune system.

Worms may be unwelcome in your cat's gastrointestinal tract, but that doesn't mean they are dangerous, unless they are allowed to overstay their visit. Unfortunately, that welcome can be as little as a few days for some cats, especially kittens, whose immune system and fragile state make them very vulnerable to a worm infestation. Worms that stay too long can rob your cat of nutrition and leave him fatigued and ill, and in some cases even threaten his life. Therefore, worms are unwelcome visitors that need to leave, and soon. Regardless of

how the visitors arrived—whether they were ingested by licking fleas or from other cats or by some other means—you can
eliminate them safely.

First, however, let's meet the enemies and how to recognize them.

WHICH WORMS AFFECT CATS?

Cats can be infected by several different intestinal worms,
and the most common invaders are roundworms, tapeworms, and coccidia. Here's a brief "bio" of each of these
pesky creatures so you can better understand the critters
with which you may have to deal.

Roundworms

Despite their name, roundworms (*Toxascaris leonina, Toxo-
cara cati*) look like pieces of white thread that are about
three to five inches long when they are adults. Roundworms
are the most common parasite to take up residence in a cat's
intestinal tract, affecting anywhere from 25 percent to 75
percent of cats, and sometimes an even higher percentage of
kittens. A cat can become infested with roundworms if she
eats a bird or rodent that has roundworm larvae in its tissues
(has your indoor cat caught a mouse lately?) or by consuming roundworm eggs from another cat's feces, because
roundworm eggs are passed in the stool of infected cats.
Kittens can become infected from their mother's milk. *Tox-
ocara cati* can be transmitted through the milk, but not
Toxascaris leonina.

Veterinarians can detect roundworms during microscopic examination of a stool sample. A roundworm infestation can be life threatening if an excessive number of the
parasites manage to block the intestinal tract. Kittens are at
greatest risk for this problem, so it's especially critical to
treat them promptly. Roundworms are usually less serious
in adult cats, but the pests still should be eliminated as soon

as possible. Pet parents should be sure to treat their cat if roundworms are discovered.

Clues that your cat may have roundworms include "strings" in the stool or vomit, a dull coat, lack of appetite, diarrhea, and a distended abdomen.

Hookworms

Although less common than roundworms, hookworms (*Ancylostoma tubaeforme*, *A. braziliense*, and *Uncinaria stenocephala*) are believed to infect between 10 and 60 percent of cats in North America. Hookworms are so named because they have tiny "hooks" or grasping structures that allow them to latch onto the intestinal wall of your cat. This hooking ability can cause cats to lose blood where the worms attach and result in feces that are tarry and black with blood. Cats who lose too much blood can become anemic and may even die if they are not treated. Other symptoms may include pale gums, weakness, dull and/or dry coat, and, in kittens, stunted growth.

Adult cats usually get hookworms by eating an infected rodent. Kittens, however, usually get them from their mother. Once the larvae are inside your cat, they move into the lungs and then the intestinal tract, where they develop into adult worms. As adults, hookworms are usually less than ½ inch long, and because they are so small they are usually not visible in the stools of infected cats. Hookworms are hardy and can live in your cat's intestinal tract for her entire life. Your veterinarian can identify hookworms by examining fecal samples from your cat.

Tapeworms

"Mommy, Tiger has pieces of rice near her tail." That's how one pet parent learned that her five-year-old Siamese mix had tapeworms. The rice to which the little girl was referring were actually segments of a tapeworm that had broken off from the adult tapeworm, which had its head attached to

Tiger's intestinal wall. As the segments at the tail end of a tapeworm mature, they break away and leave the cat's body in its feces.

Although noticing "rice" near your cat's tail is one way to discover tapeworms, another is by microscopic examination of stool samples. Tiger likely became infected by eating an infected mouse or swallowing infected fleas while he groomed himself. The different tapeworms a veterinarian may find in Tiger include *Dipylidium caninum*, *Echinococcus granulosus* and *E. multilocularis*, *Diphyllobothrium latum*, *Spirometra mansonoides*, and *Taenia* species.

DIAGNOSING WORMS

A veterinarian can diagnose the specific type of worm that may be infecting your cat by doing a microscopic examination of one or more stool samples. More than one fecal sample may be necessary, because even though your cat may have worms, there is no guarantee the sample you bring to your veterinarian will contain the eggs, larvae, or adult worms to prove it. Adult hookworms, for example, usually are not found in feces. Vomiting is another possible sign of the presence of worms, and you may see worms in the vomit.

CONVENTIONAL TREATMENT

When treating your cat for intestinal worms, typically there are two things you need to consider: ridding your cat of the worms themselves, and attacking the cause. That means if fleas are a possible cause or contributor to your cat's case of intestinal worms, you will need to get rid of the fleas as well, or else you will have two problems: a continuing case of fleas and the return of the worms. Veterinarians typically recommend a number of dewormer medications as treatment, depending on which worms they identify in your cat's stool and/or vomit. Here is a list of medications you may be prescribed for your cat:

- **Emodepside/praziquantel** (e.g., Profender) for roundworms, tapeworms, and hookworms; also treats ear mites and heartworm. This is a topical medication and may cause irritation and/or hair loss at or near the application site.
- **Epsiprantel** (e.g., Cestex) for tapeworms. In rare cases this dewormer can cause diarrhea or vomiting.
- **Imidacloprid/moxidectin** (e.g., Advantage Multi for Cats) for roundworms and hookworms; also treats heartworm, ear mites and fleas. This is a topical medication that may cause scratching or other skin irritation. Rarely, cats experience drooling, sleepiness, increased drinking, or behavior changes.
- **Milbemycin oxime** (e.g., Interceptor) for roundworms. Side effects are rare but may include anorexia (loss of appetite), depression, diarrhea, excessive salivation, lethargy, seizures, staggering, vomiting, and weakness.
- **Piperazine salts** (e.g., Sergeant's Worm Away) for for roundworms. Also available over the counter. May cause muscle tremors, nausea, and vomiting.
- **Praziquantel** (e.g., Droncit Feline Cestocide) for tapeworms. Side effects are rare but may cause diarrhea, sedation, staggering, and vomiting.
- **Pyrantel pamoate/praziquantel** (e.g., Drontal) for roundworms and tapeworms; also heartworm. Side effects associated with pyrantel pamoate are rare, and vomiting occurs infrequently. Praziquantel also rarely causes side effects, but they may include diarrhea, sedation, staggering, and vomiting.
- **Selamectin** (e.g., Revolution) for roundworms; also treats ear mites and fleas. This is a topical medication that may cause irritation or loss of hair at the application site. Contact your veterinarian if your

cat experiencing diarrhea, drooling, incoordination, rapid breathing, or vomiting.

HOME REMEDIES

If you are reluctant to give poison to your cat to kill worm eggs, larvae, and adults, you're not alone. Several natural remedies can be used to help achieve and maintain a healthy, balanced intestinal tract as well as prevent and treat worms in cats. Keep in mind, however, that a heavy worm infestation will likely require medication, although home remedies may be used in addition to and as a future preventive step. Home remedies also typically take longer to work than do medications. Consult your veterinarian.

Probiotics

Probiotics are good or friendly bacteria that can help restore your cat's intestinal tract to a healthier balance and thus may help rid your cat's body of intestinal worms and other harmful organisms. Thus far there are no studies showing probiotics to be effective in managing intestinal worms in cats, but some limited work has been done showing that beneficial bacteria can inhibit the development of certain parasites, including giardia, protozoa that infect the intestinal tract in cats.

The harmful effects of intestinal worms on a cat's intestinal tract and ability to absorb nutrients may be helped with the addition of probiotics. The main probiotics are lactobacillus (e.g., *Lactobacillus acidophilus*, *L. bulgaricus*, *L. reuteri*, *L. thermophilus*), bifidobacterium (e.g., *Bifidobacterium animalis*, *B. bifidus*, *B. lactis*, *B. longum*), enterococcus (e.g., *Enterococcus faecium*), and streptococcus (e.g., *Streptococcus thermophilus*). When choosing a probiotic supplement for your cat, look for those that contain a variety of species and strains for optimal benefit.

Dosages of probiotics are given in CFUs—colony forming units—and are expressed in millions or billions of live cells. The exact dose for your cat is not as important as giving probiotics regularly so the good bacteria can help keep bad bacteria at bay and maintain a healthy environment in your cat's intestinal tract to prevent further invasion by intestinal worms. A suggested dose for cats who have worms is at least 2 to 3 billion CFUs daily. You can reduce the dose by half once the worms have been eliminated. If you are giving your cat prescribed dewormers, probiotics can be used safely along with the drugs, and in fact are recommended.

Pumpkin Seeds

You can use ground pumpkin seeds (*Cucurbita pepo*) either alone or, for best results, along with wheat germ oil and ground figs to treat and prevent tapeworms. Pumpkin seeds are effective because they contain cucurbitin, an amino acid that can help kill tapeworms. To give your cat pumpkin seeds, you will need a food processor or coffee grinder so you can thoroughly grind fresh, raw pumpkin seeds. The most potent pumpkin seeds are those that are ground daily, but you can prepare a batch and freeze the powder in an airtight container so no moisture gets in and reduces the potency.

After you rinse and thoroughly dry raw, fresh pumpkin seeds, grind them and add ¼ teaspoon to your cat's canned food daily, mixing well. If you feed your cat twice a day, divide the dose. This is a better approach, as some cats resist anything new in their food. Feed ground pumpkin seeds to your cat for sixty days to get rid of tapeworms.

One way to enhance the ability of ground pumpkin seeds to eliminate tapeworms is to add ¼ teaspoon of wheat germ oil to your cat's food as well. If you want to help prevent the return of tapeworms, continue giving your cat the wheat germ oil after the sixty days of pumpkin seed treatment. Another way to boost your efforts to rid your cat of tapeworms is to add ¼ teaspoon of ground figs to your cat's food in addition to the pumpkin seed and wheat germ oil. Grind chopped dried figs in a food processor or coffee grinder.

Wormwood

The very name of this herb suggests it can be used to treat worms, and indeed it is a traditional remedy for getting rid of roundworms and tapeworms in pets as well as in people. However, wormwood (*Artemisia absinthium*) is potent and should be used with caution. It contains volatile oil (primarily thujone), absinthum, and tannins that can be irritating and even harmful to the kidneys, so wormwood should be used only with the advice of your veterinarian. You can purchase wormwood tincture, which is likely the easiest way to give this herb to your cat. Although wormwood can be effective, it also has a bitter taste, and so many cats will not accept it. The maximum dose for a cat is 1/2 teaspoon daily, which you can divide into several doses along with wet food. Do not give your cat wormwood for more than three consecutive days.

Other Home Remedies

There are a variety of natural wormers on the market that contain a combination of herbs marketed as being beneficial in eliminating intestinal parasites from cats. Talk to your veterinarian before using any of these products. Typically these formulas contain wormwood along with other ingredients that may include those listed below.

- **Black walnut.** The unripe hulls of black walnuts are used to manage parasites. This is a folk remedy and thus far no scientific studies have proven it works against intestinal parasites in cats. However, it is sometimes included in herbal dewormers.
- **Cloves (*Eugenia caryophyllata*).** This spice has antiparasitic and bactericidal properties.
- **Goldenseal.** This herb contains berberine, which has been shown to help fight parasites.

- **Herb of grace (*Ruta graveolens*).** This is an ancient herb (also known as common rue) with a long history of use to fight rheumatism and intestinal worms, among other ills. Although I couldn't find any scientific evidence to back up the claims, it has anecdotal evidence on its side.
- **Neem (*Azadirachta indica*).** At least one scientific study shows neem seed extract to be effective in fighting fleas in cats. Since worms and fleas share an intimate relationship, it's not unusual to see neem in products used to fight worms.

In addition, many herbal dewormers also contain an herbal laxative, which can help your cat eliminate the parasites, but also may cause loose stools. Therefore, it is recommended you avoid products that contain laxatives, such as cascara sagrada bark and senna.

Chapter 15

Kidney Disease

Among aging cats, kidney disease, also known as kidney failure or chronic renal disease, is a major health problem and the cause of death second only to feline leukemia. It's estimated that 8 percent of cats who are ten years or older have kidney failure, although the disease can affect younger cats as well.

One reason kidney failure is so serious is that it is often insidious. It can seem to appear overnight, when in fact the factors responsible for the organ problems can develop over months, even years, with no apparent symptoms. Yet, when symptoms do appear, the kidney damage has been done: Once the kidneys have been harmed, they cannot be repaired. If, however, it's a case of acute kidney failure, which I discuss in this chapter, you may be able to prevent kidney damage if you catch it in time.

Despite the seriousness of kidney failure, there is much pet parents and veterinarians can do to help affected cats enjoy a good quality of life; in fact, that's the main message in this chapter. Before we launch into how to care for a cat who has kidney failure, it helps to understand what kidney failure is and how the kidneys work.

WHAT IS KIDNEY FAILURE?

The term "kidney failure," even though it is commonly used, is actually somewhat of a misnomer. Kidney failure in cats refers to a progressive decline in healthy kidney function, which can be caused by a number of different reasons ranging from genetics to urinary tract diseases or other ailments to trauma. Therefore, cats are said to have kidney failure, yet their kidneys still function, but not the way they should.

The main job of the kidneys is to filter and process waste from the blood, as well as to regulate blood and water levels in the body. These functions are compromised in cats who have kidney failure, and at the heart of the problem is the deterioration of tiny structures in the kidneys called nephrons, which are responsible for these tasks. The bad (and good) thing about a cat's kidneys is that they are so efficient, signs of kidney failure don't usually appear until 70 percent of the nephrons have been damaged. Once nephrons have been damaged, they cannot be repaired, but the remaining nephrons can be nurtured.

As the kidneys lose their ability to remove waste materials from a cat's blood, poisons accumulate in the blood and eventually cause signs and symptoms of uremic poisoning. The sooner pet parents and veterinarians recognize indications of kidney failure, the faster treatment can begin and the better chance a cat has to live a good life.

TYPES AND CAUSES OF KIDNEY FAILURE

Cats are susceptible to two different types of kidney failure: acute and chronic. Because the causes, symptoms, and treatments differ between the two types, let's look at each one separately.

Acute Kidney Failure

Acute kidney failure refers to a sudden or abrupt failure of the kidneys to function properly and is much less common than chronic kidney failure. This type of kidney failure causes an accumulation of waste products and other poisons in the bloodstream, dehydration, and imbalances in electrolyte levels (essential nutrients such as calcium, sodium, and magnesium) and the acid-base ratio in the bloodstream.

Acute kidney failure can be caused by a variety of factors. One of the more common causes is poisoning, especially with antifreeze (ethylene glycol, which has a taste that can attract cats) and rat poison. Other causes can include:

- An obstructed urethra, which may be associated with feline lower urinary tract disease
- Shock related to a sudden loss of blood or dehydration
- Trauma or injury to the abdomen and/or pelvic area
- Snake- or insect bite and venom
- Blood clotting disorder
- Heart failure associated with chronic low blood pressure
- Use of medications such as antibiotics of nonsteroidal anti-inflammatory drugs
- Ingestion of heavy metals such as mercury, lead, and arsenic
- Presence of feline infectious peritonitis, pyelonephritis, or a bacterial infection of the kidney.

The more quickly and aggressively a cat with acute kidney failure is diagnosed and treated, the better chance you have of stopping any further destruction of nephrons and reversing the disease. Delayed treatment can lead to death. Cats who have an infection have a better prognosis than do those who have been poisoned.

Chronic Kidney Failure

Chronic kidney failure is much more common than the acute variety and is often seen in older cats. Although experts have assembled a list of possible causes for chronic kidney failure, the truth is that for many older cats, the exact cause of the kidney failure is never identified. A growing number of veterinarians and companion animal experts believe that a poor diet, specifically one based on dry cat food, is a significant contributor to chronic kidney failure. Among them is Elizabeth M. Hodgkins, DVM, who has stated that cats who consume a dry food diet year after year eat their way into "a chronic state of dehydration" and lay the foundation for kidney failure.

That said, here is a list of causes of chronic kidney failure. You may notice that some of these causes are also associated with acute kidney failure.

- Advancing age, as most elderly cats have some degree of kidney dysfunction
- Infectious diseases, such as feline leukemia and feline infectious peritonitis
- Long-term use of antibiotics (e.g., amphotericin B, gentamicin, kanamycin, polymyxin B), especially when given in high doses
- Exposure to heavy metals
- Nephritis (inflammation of the nephrons) and nephrosis (a noninflammatory, degenerative disease that attacks the canals in the kidney)
- Use of nonsteroidal anti-inflammatory drugs, especially if taken when a cat is experiencing low blood pressure
- Hyperthyroidism, which often occurs along with chronic kidney failure

DOES MY CAT HAVE KIDNEY FAILURE?

Symptoms of acute kidney failure and chronic kidney failure are somewhat different, so it pays to know them both.

Cats who experience acute kidney failure may have had recent exposure to poison or have had an illness, trauma, or surgery. Symptoms of acute kidney failure usually include:

- Sudden loss of appetite
- Listlessness
- Disorientation
- Vomiting, which may contain blood

- Diarrhea, which may contain blood
- Foul or unusual breath odor
- Seizures
- Sudden change in urination habits: peeing more often or not at all.

Cats who have chronic kidney failure typically do not display symptoms until the damage to the nephrons is irreversible. Symptoms of chronic kidney failure include the following:

- Increase in the frequency of urination. (Sometimes cats begin to urinate outside of their litter box.)
- Increase in water consumption
- Drooling
- Dehydration
- Weight loss
- Bad breath (may smell like ammonia)
- Bladder or kidney infections
- Apathy, lethargy
- Dry haircoat
- Brown tongue
- Gum and tongue ulcers
- Vomiting
- Diarrhea
- Anemia
- Gastrointestinal bleeding
- Urination stops, coma (late stage).

DIAGNOSING KIDNEY FAILURE

Cats who have acute kidney failure are typically in a life-threatening situation, so a quick, accurate diagnosis is critical. Any information you and other pet parents can provide—including the cat's exposure to toxins, recent medical procedures and/or medication use, plus any symptoms and behaviors they have noticed recently—can be helpful for the veterinarian. In cats who have acute kidney failure, veterinarians often find painful, enlarged kidneys when they perform their physical examination. Tests that may be ordered include one or more of the following:

- Serum biochemistry profile, which provides a wealth of information on levels of critical substances in serum (the liquid portion of the blood), such as kidney proteins, calcium, electrolytes (e.g., sodium, chloride, potassium, magnesium), enzymes, cholesterol, glucose, and bilirubin
- Urinalysis, which will show if the kidneys are able to filter and concentrate the urine
- X-rays of the abdomen
- Ultrasound
- Ethylene glycol test
- Blood tests for signs of infections
- Fine-needle aspiration or biopsy of the kidneys.

CONVENTIONAL TREATMENT

A conventional treatment approach depends on the type of kidney failure. The main treatment goals in cats who have acute kidney failure are to eliminate the poison or infection in the system as quickly as possible, rehydrate, and rebalance the electrolytes and the acid-base ratio. It is possible to reverse acute kidney failure if a veterinarian can stop the cause before it damages the nephrons permanently. If your cat has ingested something toxic, she may need to have her stomach emptied and then be treated with activated charcoal to prevent further poisoning. In severe cases, dialysis may be necessary, but this treatment is not widely available and is extremely expensive. Standard treatment involves giving intravenous fluids for at least twenty-four hours and up to four days. It is critical to be sure your cat gets lots of water to make up for the large amount of fluids being lost. If your cat experiences persistent vomiting, nutritional therapy may be necessary as well.

Treatment of chronic kidney failure involves a permanent change in diet for a cat. Cats who have chronic kidney failure still need a diet that is high in protein, but the protein sources need to be chosen carefully because most animal protein is high in phosphorus (phosphate), a mineral that is harmful to the kidneys of a cat who had chronic kidney failure.

An option is for your cat to take a phosphorus binder, such as aluminum hydroxide salt (Amphojel) or Epakitin, which contains lactose, calcium carbonate, chitosan, and hydrolyzed soy protein. Cats who have chronic kidney disease absorb more phosphorus than do healthy cats, which damages their kidneys. These phosphorus binders help prevent the absorption of phosphorus. Although ideally they should be used along with a low-phosphorus diet, they can also be used along with regular cat food when cats refuse to eat foods that are low in phosphorus. See more about diet for chronic kidney disease under "Home Remedies" below.

Veterinarians may prescribe medications for cats who temporarily experience vomiting, including famotidine, omeprazole, or ranitidine. Cats who have high blood pressure may require medications to bring it down, while the development of anemia may require the use of erythropoietin, but this treatment is usually reserved for cats who have long-term kidney failure. In some cases, cats become dehydrated and require hospitalization to replace fluids.

HOME REMEDIES

Diet is critical when it comes to treating a cat who has kidney failure. A carefully planned dietary plan can be enhanced by several home remedies that include nutritional and herbal supplements.

Diet

For years, the diet mantra for cats with chronic kidney failure has been "low protein, low phosphorus," but fortunately part of that tune is changing, and the result is healthier cats. The part to keep is "low phosphorus," because too much phosphorus can cause a further decline in kidney function. However, cats are carnivores, whether they have chronic kidney failure or not, and they need high amounts of protein to thrive. Therefore, placing a cat whose kidneys are failing on a protein-restricted diet, which is still a common practice, is not wise. Dr. Hodgkins notes that while a protein-restricted diet has become very popular over recent decades, "ironically, this switch to a low-protein diet is misguided, and may cause a great deal more harm than good" in cats with chronic kidney failure.

Dr. Hodgkins has pointed out that cats who are deprived of sufficient protein cannot initiate their own natural healing process or produce enough energy to survive. Thus, a pet parent who thinks she is doing the right thing by placing her ill cat on a low-protein diet may end up blaming the disease for their cat's demise instead of the diet. Says Hodgkins, when such a cat does not get the protein it needs, "it wastes away and dies, and CRD [chronic renal disease] gets all the blame. There have never been any scientific studies showing long-term benefits from a reduction in dietary protein that justify this restriction, compared to low-carbohydrate diets with higher protein, in the cat with CRD."

So, what should you feed your cat if she has chronic kidney disease? One way to face the challenge of providing adequate protein but low phosphorus is to add cooked egg whites to your cat's high-quality canned or homemade food. Egg whites are a great source of protein and also contain no phosphate, so it helps dilute the phosphorus in the food, according to Hodgkins. Another way to provide high protein without worrying about phosphorus is to give your cat a phosphate binder, which you can add to your cat's regular wet food diet to eliminate a significant amount of phosphorus from the food.

Dandelion

Diuretic herbs are plants that have the ability to prompt the kidneys to produce urine, which then allows the body to eliminate waste. One common diuretic herb is dandelion. Although you may think of the dandelion as a weed, it is a well-tolerated herbal diuretic, and you can add dandelion tincture to your cat's water or food to promote urination. Try adding one or two drops to her food or water daily.

Vitamins, Minerals and Enzymes

Cats who have chronic kidney failure can lose a large amount of several important vitamins and minerals in their urine, including the family of the water-soluble B vitamins, potassium, vitamin D, and calcitriol (calcium). Talk to your veterinarian about the need for your cat to take a B-complex supplement as well as supplements of each of these nutrients.

Also consider supplements of taurine. A suggested dose is 250 to 500 mg twice daily. This amino acid and enzyme plays an important role in the regulating the function of the kidneys. Because cats cannot make their own taurine from other amino acids as dogs and people can, they must get it from their diet. If you are feeding your cat a homemade diet, be sure you are including ingredients that are high in taurine (e.g., beef, beef liver, chicken, fish, shrimp, and nutritional yeast).

Feeding Tricks

Many cats who have chronic kidney failure are problem eaters. In fact, it's not uncommon for them to lose all interest in food. Although in some cases this means the cat is ready to make his transition, typically it simply means the cat needs to be encouraged to eat and will have a reasonably good quality of life if you can somehow encourage him to eat. Time is of the essence, however, as cats in this condition who will not eat can decline rapidly. So, here are a few feeding tricks and tips some pet parents have found to be helpful in getting a cat with chronic kidney failure to eat.

✓ **Raise the bowl.** You can do it easily by placing bricks, a box, books, or anything that will safely and securely raise the bowl up to mouth level. Some cats respond well to this simple change.

✓ **Warm the food.** Warm food has more taste, and it is closer to body temperature than cold food. Either serve at room temperature or heat refrigerated food in a microwave for a few seconds. If you microwave, be sure to stir the food before serving and make sure there are no hot spots.

✓ **Serve food when sleepy.** That means when your cat is sleepy, not you! If your cat is not fully awake and smells food, she may start eating without thinking about it, or at least that appears to be why this trick sometimes works.

✓ **Provide homemade food.** Homemade recipes provide new smells and tastes that may entice your cat to eat. One simple favorite is homemade chicken or turkey broth, made by boiling a chicken or turkey parts in water. (Do not add salt or seasonings to the water, and do not use fowl that has added broth.) When cooled to room temperature, homemade broth provides nutrients and much-needed fluids, and many cats seem to really enjoy homemade broth. You can also use the broth to put on other food to encourage your cat to eat.

✓ **Try a new feeding location.** A food bowl placed in a different location in the house may trick your cat into eating. Is the bowl now near her favorite place to sleep? Then move it into another room. Also try dividing up the food and placing it into three or four bowls and putting them around the house.

✓ **Feed your cat by hand.** Yes, this takes time, but sometimes this is the only way a cat will eat. Of course, try all the other suggestions as well. Feeding by hand is usually a last resort.

✓ **Add new flavors.** Sometimes it helps to add some new flavorings to the food, such as water from tuna packed in water, Parmesan cheese, or dried bonito flakes.

Chapter 16
Obesity

Chubby kittens are cute, but that baby fat, just like in human babies, can morph into excess weight in adulthood and an overweight or obese—and unhealthy—adult cat. Although we've grown accustomed to the well-fed cat look popularized by fictional cats like Garfield, the fact is, fat is neither funny nor smart.

According to a report released by the Association of Pet Obesity Prevention (APOP) in February 2011, 53 percent of cats in the United States are either overweight or obese, which translates into roughly 50 million kitties. Do these numbers sound familiar? That's because more than half of the adults in the United States—actually, closer to about 65 percent—also are overweight or obese. The cats are catching up with their pet parents, who, in fact, are a major part of the problem.

Cats don't get fat by themselves. When was the last time you saw an obese feral cat? How about a cat who drove himself to the grocery store and bought a cart full of cat treats or one who filled his own bowl? Cats become overweight and obese because people feed them too much food, and often poor-quality food to boot. Pet parents need to recognize when their cat is carrying too much weight and then take the necessary steps to make sure the weight comes off safely and slowly. Overweight and obese cats are at high risk of serious health problems, such as diabetes, arthritis, and kidney disease, and preventing these diseases begins with a nutritious diet that provides high-quality calories that do not pack on extra pounds.

IS MY CAT OVERWEIGHT?

Congratulations! If you are questioning whether your cat is overweight or obese, that's an important first step, because many pet parents believe—or want to believe—that a chubby cat is a happy, healthy cat, or that their cat is not overweight. To help you determine if your cat is overweight, follow these simple steps. These steps are best done while your cat is standing.

- ✓ **Feel your cat's ribs.** You should feel a slight amount of fat on the ribs, but still easily feel each rib individually. If you can see the ribs, your cat is underweight, and if you can't feel them at all unless you press hard (which you don't want to do), then your cat is overweight.
- ✓ **Feel the base of your cat's tail.** You might call this the tailbone area. A slight, smooth pad of fat should be over this area. If the bones stick out, your cat is too thin, but if you can't feel any bones at all, then kitty is too fat.
- ✓ **Check other sites.** Feel your cat's hips, spine, and shoulders. All of these areas should be covered by a slight pad of fat. If you can see the bones or easily feel them in any of these areas, then your cat is too thin. If you find yourself fishing for the bones, then your cat is overweight.
- ✓ **Look at your cat from above.** View your standing cat from above and look for the waistline. A normal weight can has a definite waistline, while a cat who is too thin will have an hourglass figure. An overweight cat will have no waistline or a pudginess where the waistline should be, which is behind the ribs.
- ✓ **Check the skin.** If you pick up your cat's skin anywhere on his body, you should not feel a thick pad of fat underneath.

✓ **Do a side view.** Cats of a healthy weight have a tucked in abdomen, which is the area just behind the ribs. Cats who are overweight have no tuck. Note that many cats have an apron, which is loose skin that hangs on the underside of the abdomen. This is not fat nor a sign your cat is overweight. However, don't fool yourself into believing a big belly is really an apron. If you follow all the steps presented here and answer honestly, you'll have your answer.

DIAGNOSING OBESITY

The steps outlined under "Is My Cat Overweight?" above are similar to the ones veterinarians typically take to determine if a cat is overweight. Before you decide to help your cat shed some of those extra pounds, it's critical that your veterinarian determine if there are medical reasons why your cat is carrying extra pounds. Therefore, a thorough physical examination, accurate recording of weight, and blood chemistry should be done, including a thyroid hormone test, to make sure your cat is not suffering from hypothyroidism (inadequate thyroid hormone production, which promotes weight gain) or diabetes, or has any condition that could be contributing to the problem. In addition, it's important to know if your cat has another health conditions that may interfere with or influence whatever weight-loss program you want to follow. If your cat is found to be in good health except for the weight problem, then it's time to set up a weight loss program.

CONVENTIONAL TREATMENT

Veterinarians faced with an overweight or obese cat typically recommend that pet parents place the kitty on a prescription weight management food (dry or canned, although more are recommending wet food) and help the cat get more exercise. However, many of the so-called diet or weight management foods are too high in fiber, which means they are also too high in carbohydrates. All cats, overweight or normal weight, need high protein and low carbs.

Beware, however, of low-carbohydrate dry cat foods, which are high in calories. This leaves high-protein, low-carbohydrate canned food as your best choice if you elect to stay with commercial foods. If you now feeding your cat dry food and you make a gradual change to a high-quality wet food, the weight should come off slowly and steadily. If it does not, then you may need to reduce the portions slightly. And don't forget the all-important exercise factor!

Because diet and exercise are really home remedy approaches, the remainder of the recommendations are offered under that heading.

HOME REMEDIES

Helping your kitty lose a few pounds is a labor of love, and one that will pay off in big rewards for both your cat and you.

How to Help Your Cat Lose Weight

- ✓ **Banish free feeding.** All food, all the time: That's the American way and a recipe for obesity. Since the food offered at free feeding is usually dry food, the problem is even worse, since dry cat food (even high-quality brands) is not a healthy choice for cats, primary because of its high carbohydrate content. As discussed in chapter 1, "Basic Nutrition: What Your Cat Needs," cats require only about 5 percent of their calories to come from carbohydrates, yet dry cat food provides 20, 30, even 50 percent and more in some cases.

- ✓ **Offer several small meals.** Determine how much food your cat needs per day (see chapter 1) and then divide that amount into two to four servings of canned food, homemade food, or a mixture of the two.

✓ **Don't feed a beggar.** If your cat is begging—perhaps by vocalizing, butting you with her head, following you around the house—don't give in. If you relent and give your cat a food treat, then you have reinforced the behavior, and you can expect more vocalizing, butting, and following. Instead, when your cat begs, give him attention: scratching behind the ears, combing or brushing, playing with a toy, a belly rub. Remember, these are all no-calorie treats!

✓ **Ignore the labels.** Cat food labels provide feeding instructions that generally are designed to make sure you buy more cat food and feed your cat more food than she needs, especially if she is being fed dry food. The feeding instructions on canned food are also culprits. Generally, you can follow the feeding suggestions presented in chapter 1, but always remember that every cat is different, and you will need to monitor your cat's food intake and weight throughout this weight loss process.

✓ **Exercise.** No, you don't need to break out the kitty jogging suit, but you can encourage your sedentary cat to be more physical. Some cat breeds are inherently more active than others, such as Abyssinians and Bengals, but for the most part cats need to be encouraged to move, especially older and overweight cats. (See "Cat Exercise Tips" on page 182 for a bunch of ideas to keep your cat moving!)

✓ **Weigh in.** Establish your cat's starting weight (either at your veterinarian's office or at home using an accurate scale, preferably a digital) and then weigh in every three to four weeks to keep track of your progress. If there is no change after three to four weeks, then make adjustments to the amount of food you are feeding and/or the calories you are feeding.

✓ **Be patient.** It took time for the weight to accumulate, so it will take time for it to come off. A cat that is forced to lose weight too rapidly can develop a potentially deadly condition called hepatic lipidosis. As a guide, a 15-pound cat, who should weigh about 12 pounds, should not lose more than ½ pound every four weeks (which is 2 ounces per week) to avoid complications such as hepatic lipidosis.

✓ **Establish a maintenance diet.** Once your cat has reached her ideal weight (hooray!), keep an eye on her weight and her food intake and determine how much food she needs to maintain her new figure and improved health.

✓ **Offer high-protein, moderate-fat, very-low-carb food.** A high-protein diet is essential for an overweight cat to lose weight. Although there are still some pet experts who subscribe to feeding a fat cat a high-fiber diet, this approach has largely been put in the closet by feline nutrition experts, since cats do not do well with too many carbohydrates, and fiber is carbs.

Canned cat food contains about 20 to 40 calories per ounce. You can use the calculator presented in chapter 1 to help you determine how many calories are in the canned cat food on your pantry shelf. If you are using homemade recipes from your veterinarian or from other sources, look for those that provide calorie counts. But how many calories should you be feeding your chubby cat?

There's a formula offered by Lisa A. Pierson, DVM, on her Web site, you can follow to help you make that determination. First, what is your cat's ideal weight? If female, 10 to 11 pounds is optimal; if male, 11 to 13 pounds. Then use this formula to figure out how many calories to feed your cat:

$13.6 \times XX$ pounds $+ 70 =$ calories per day

For example: if your female cat weighs 15 pounds and you want to get her to a healthy 11 pounds, use this formula:

$$(13.6 \times 11 \text{ pounds}) + 70 = 219.6 \text{ calories per day}$$

The 219 calories per day is a starting point, because it is likely too high to help your cat lose weight. However, if you feed your cat 219 calories per day for two weeks and she has not lost any weight after two weeks, reduce the number of calories per day by 20 percent. This is a general suggestion: Every cat metabolizes food at a different rate, so it's important to weigh your cat every three to four days to make sure he is not losing weight too rapidly or not losing weight at all.

A safe rate of weight loss for a cat is 1 to 2 percent of his current body weight per week. Just like people, cats reach a plateau during their weight-loss efforts. Therefore, as your cat loses weight, the number of ounces lost per week decline, but don't lose the faith! With persistence and patience you and your kitty will reach your goal.

Homemade Recipes

If you are making your own homemade cat food, choose recipes that provide calorie counts, or you can determine the calorie count yourself (or fairly accurately) by using a calorie counter, which are offered by many Web sites and books. Obviously, the fewer ingredients in the recipe, the easier it will be to determine the calorie count. For example, let's break down this simple recipe, which is designed to feed a 10-pound cat two servings per day for three days.

Simple Chicken Delight

2 cups chopped lean chicken thigh, meat only (about 500 calories)
4 tsp ground flaxseed (50 calories)
2 Tbs mashed cooked broccoli or carrots (6 calories)

2 Tbs brown rice (26 calories)
2 multivitamin/mineral supplements w/taurine

This recipe provides approximately 194 calories per day (582 total calories for the recipe divided by 3 days).

Cat Exercise Tips

If your cat is home alone all day, then she has no reason to move around (except to hit the food bowl filled with dry kibble—a big no-no!). Although you may want to spend lots of time playing with your cat, you may not have that luxury. Any time you do spend with kitty, however, is important because it allows you to bond as well as provide physical activity. Since the latter is the purpose here, here are some cat exercise tips. Recruit other family members to help with the exercise as well.

- ✓ **Consider adopting another cat so they can play together.** Obviously there is additional expense having more than one cat, but it is an option that can help resolve the problem of boredom and an accompanying weight issue, while a benefit is the additional pleasure of sharing your time with two kitties.
- ✓ **Separate the litter box from the feeding area.** In fact, the farther away these two objects are from each other, the better, because then your cat is required to walk from one to the other. If you can place the litter box and feeding bowl on separate floors, thus requiring your cat to climb stairs, that's even better.
- ✓ **Provide commercial toys.** Not every cat likes toys, especially as they get older, but there are so many on the market, it's worth a try. Movement is critical: Cats like objects that mimic prey in nature, so a ball or toy that moves, an object on the end of a string or fishing-pole-like object, or a rolling object may spark some interest.

✓ **Devise homemade toys.** These ideas are cost-effective and can be entertaining. For example, place open brown paper grocery bags or medium-sized cardboard boxes around the house. Many cats can entertain themselves by darting in and out of bags and boxes. Suspend feathers, bells, or other small objects from string that are tied to doorknobs or other convenient places. A tightly wadded ball of aluminum foil or paper can be a great "soccer ball" for your cat. Just be sure your cat cannot swallow or become entangled in whatever toy you provide.

✓ **Try techno-toys.** Let your cat enter the techno-age by providing a remote controlled toy, such as a remote-controlled mouse, or let him chase a laser pointer or a small flashlight beam in a dark room. Be sure to never direct the light beam into your cat's eyes.

✓ **Provide climbing posts.** Cats like heights and to climb, so commercially available scratching/climbing posts and cat trees can provide an opportunity for exercise. Some of these trees have sleeping areas that your cat may enjoy.

✓ **Rotate the toys.** Kids get bored with toys, and so do cats. A good way to avoid boredom is to rotate the toys: Leave out certain toys for a day or two, then put them away and replace them with others.

✓ **Try stimulating herb toys.** These include toys that contain either dried catnip or valerian root. I provide a fuller explanation of both below (see "Valerian" and "Catnip").

L-carnitine

Consider giving your cat a supplement of the amino acid L-carnitine. This amino acid is found in meat and plays a key role in transforming fat into glucose (sugar), which means more energy and less weight for your cat. A study published in the *Journal of Veterinary Internal Medicine*, for example, reported on twenty-four obese cats who were put on a reduced-calorie diet (i.e., calorie intake was limited to 60 percent of their maintenance calorie needs, or 60 calories/kg). Fourteen of the cats also received a 250 mg per day of L-carnitine supplement in their food. The study lasted eighteen weeks, and although cats in both test groups lost weight, those who received L-carnitine lost weight faster. It's important to note that while the cats who received L-carnitine lost weight faster, they did not lose weight *too* rapidly, which can be dangerous. The combination of a low-calorie diet and the L-carnitine resulted in a safe level of weight loss, which was about 20 percent of body weight over an eighteen-week period.

Valerian

Valerian (*Valeriana officinalis*) is an herb you might recognize as a calming remedy for humans, but in cats it has the opposite effect: It could put some zip into your kitty. That's because valerian contains a substance called actinidine, which is chemically similar to nepetalactone, the active component in catnip. Therefore, a toy that contains dried valerian can prompt your lazy cat to get up and play, and that means calories burned and a happy cat.

You can offer your cat valerian in the form of a toy stuffed with dried valerian root, or a toy that has sprayed with a valerian spray. Do *not* use valerian essential oil, because it can be toxic. To prevent your cat from getting accustomed to valerian root, offer the toy only a few times per week and watch her jump, wrestle, roll, and toss the toy for an hour or more. You can make your own toy by making a small cloth square, stuffing it with a few tablespoons of dried valerian root, and stitching it closed. You can also stuff a small sock and sew up the open end.

Catnip

Most cats love catnip (*Nepeta cataria*), a type of mint that contains an active ingredient called nepetalactone. If you have ever given your cat a catnip toy, you are probably familiar with the dreamy looks that cross your cat's face, but it's the kitten-like playful behavior that means calories are being burned. You can grow your own catnip (just be sure to keep the plants away from your cat!) and use either fresh or dried leaves to make your own catnip toys (see "Valerian" above). Whether you grow your own catnip or buy it fresh, keep the leaves, fresh or dried, in ceramic, metal, or dark glass jars with tight lids, as light and moisture can make the leaves lose their potency.

Chapter 17

Urinary Tract Problems

Urinary tract problems in cats can be referred to by many names, but basically they all boil down to one thing: Your kitty has a pee problem. Among the most common terms used to refer to urinary tract problems in cats are urinary tract infections, feline lower urinary tract disease (FLUTD), inflammation of the bladder (cystitis), urinary crystals or stones in the bladder (urolithiasis), and partial or total obstruction of the urethra. Some of these terms overlap, as I explain in this chapter, so frequently pet parents are confused about exactly what type of urinary tract problem their cat has. Hopefully this chapter will shed some light on the matter and, more importantly, how to manage it.

Urinary tract problems affect about 1 percent of adult cats and have an impact on the function and/or structure of the bladder and/or urethra (the tube that transports urine from the bladder to the outside of the body). Both male and females cats of any age can experience urinary tract problems, although these urinary difficulties tend to be more dangerous in males because they have a longer, narrower urethra, which makes it more susceptible to infection and blockage. Although urinary tract problems can often be treated easily and effectively, it's critical to note that complete obstruction of the urethra is deadly if not treated.

DOES MY CAT HAVE A URINARY TRACT PROBLEM?

Although there are many names for urinary tract disease in cats, the symptoms are the same. Often pet parents don't even realize their cat has a urinary tract problem until the disease is well advanced, but I'd like to help you avoid that situation. Therefore, it's important to familiarize yourself with the risk factors for and the symptoms of feline lower urinary tract disease so you can recognize them and be alert to your cat's problem before it becomes more serious.

First, the risk factors. Your cat:

- Is overweight
- Is middle-aged
- Uses an indoor litter box
- Eats a dry food diet (too little water and high ash and mineral content).
- Is sedentary
- Lives in a multi-cat household.

If your cat is exhibiting any of the following signs or symptoms, feline lower urinary tract disease may be the cause, so see your veterinarian. Your cat:

- Strains to urinate
- Makes frequent and/or prolonged attempts to urinate
- Experiences pain when urinating, which may be evident by crying out when he is in the litter box
- Urinates more often than usual
- Has blood in his urine
- Licks his genital area excessively
- Urinates outside the litter box, especially on smooth, cool surfaces (e.g., the bathtub, the sink, the tile floor).

If your cat is showing any of the above signs and is passing little or no urine, he likely has an obstruction, which is an emergency and requires immediate veterinary care.

TYPES AND CAUSES OF URINARY TRACT PROBLEMS

Urinary tract issues in cats can develop in several forms and can be caused by a variety of factors, even though symptoms among the forms are similar. This fact can make it a challenge for veterinarians to diagnose the problem when you bring your kitty in for a visit. Here are the main types and causes of urinary tract problems that may affect your kitty.

Diet

Before we talk about types of urinary tract problems that are also causal in nature, it's essential to address the topic of diet. A growing number of veterinarians and other companion experts recognize that diet has a major role in causing lower urinary tract disease. One of the most vocal champions of diet as a cause of pee problems in cats is Lisa A. Pierson, DVM, who states that "if your cat is on a properly hydrated diet of 100% canned food—and no dry food—you stand a very good chance of never needing to read this Web page." The Web page to which she refers is on her site Feline Urinary Tract Health: Cystitis, Urethral Obstruction, Urinary Tract Infection. (www.catinfo.org/?link-urinarytracthealth)

The point here is that cats *must* consume an adequate amount of water to avoid developing urinary tract problems. Yet the very popular and convenient dry food provides only about 5 to 10 percent water per serving, while canned food offers cats about 78 to 80 percent water on average. And because cats have a low drive to seek water (also referred to as a low thirst drive), they do not get the additional water they need to maintain a healthy urinary tract from drinking at their water bowl. Cats need water in their food, which is how they have traditionally gotten their water naturally.

Yet another problem related to dry cat food is that some pet parents leave the food out all the time (free feeding). Cats who have access to food throughout the day tend to keep eating or eat more often than they should, especially if they are indoor cats, and this habit does not allow their urine pH to become alkaline. It's best to keep alkaline levels less than 6.8, which means the body needs to accumulate a large amount of magnesium before stones are able to form.

Speaking of magnesium, the level of this mineral in cat food is believed by some experts to be a factor in urinary tract problems. This belief has led some cat food makers to formulate "special" urinary tract foods for cats that contain lower amounts of the mineral to help prevent formation of the stones. However, many cats who are given a low-magnesium diet still get urinary tract disease and recurrence as well. Magnesium does not appear to be the problem. In fact, when you consider that a cat's natural diet (in the wild) consists of a significant amount of magnesium, the folly of this way of thinking gains more credibility.

Feline Idiopathic Cystitis

Also known as interstitial cystitis, feline idiopathic cystitis (FIC) is the most common cause of lower urinary tract signs and symptoms. Veterinarians often give a diagnosis of FIC after they do a series of tests and have not found any other specific reasons why a cat is experiencing one or more of the typical symptoms of lower urinary tract disease. Thus feline idiopathic (meaning "unknown cause") cystitis is known as a diagnosis of exclusion. In fact, between 55 and 60 percent of cats who have symptoms of lower urinary tract problems are eventually diagnosed with feline idiopathic cystitis.

Although the exact causes of FIC aren't known, risk factors appear to be stress and obesity, while immune system dysfunction, viral infections, and abnormalities in the protective layer inside the bladder (the glycosaminoglycan layer) also may play a role. The things that can be stressful for a cat can range from having a dirty litter box to having to deal with a new baby or cat in the family. As a cat pet parent you are probably familiar with many of the factors that can stress out your cat!

Urolithiasis (Urinary Stones)

Sometimes tiny stones form in the urinary tract, which can cause lower urinary tract disease in your cat. The two most common types of urinary stones are struvite and calcium oxalate. A definitive diagnosis of urinary stones usually cannot be made, however, unless the cat undergoes X-rays or ultrasound. Fortunately, a special diet may eliminate struvite stones, although stubborn ones must be removed by a surgeon. Calcium oxalate stones usually must be removed by flushing the bladder with sterile fluids or, if that fails, with surgery, because they will not dissolve with a special diet.

If your cat has been diagnosed with urinary stones, chances are he will develop them again in the future. To help prevent recurrence, veterinarians often recommend changing the cat's diet.

Urethral Obstruction

Obstruction of the urethra, whether it is complete or partial, is the most serious problem that can develop in association with urinary tract function because it threatens your cat's life. Neutered male cats are at the greatest risk for urethral obstruction because they have a short, narrow urethra. If you have a female cat, however, she is not immune to urethral obstruction so it's important to pay attention to any changes in her behavior as well.

Urinary stones are one cause of urethral obstruction; another is soft urethral plugs, which are composed of minerals, cells, and proteins. Regardless of the cause of the blockage, it's critical to open up the urethra, especially if it is blocked completely and therefore is not allowing the kidneys to remove toxins from the blood or maintain the fluid and electrolyte balance in the cat's body. This is a life-or-death situation, and cats can die within twenty-four to forty-eight hours of the development of complete urethral obstruction unless the blockage is cleared.

Other Causes of Lower Urinary Tract Disease

In a small number of cases, lower urinary tract disease in cats is caused by a bacterial infection (1 to 3 percent of cases), cancer (1 percent), or trauma to or structural defects of the urethra (less than 1 percent). Another contributing factor is stress.

HOW TO REDUCE YOUR CAT'S STRESS

Did you know there appears to be a common thread between feline interstitial cystitis and interstitial cystitis in humans? That thread is stress. While stress can trigger FIC, it's also known that an emotionally stressful event often occurs before people experience lower urinary tract symptoms associated with interstitial cystitis. I won't tell you how to relieve your own stress, but here's how you can help your kitty.

- ✓ **Keep the litter box clean at all times.**
- ✓ **Allow your kitty to practice his predatory nature.** Provide places or structures to climb, scratching posts, toys to chase, and opportunities to view the outside world (a window bed is a nice touch).
- ✓ **Feed your cat on a schedule.**
- ✓ **If you need to change his food, do it very gradually over several weeks.** Include more wet food each day as you withdraw the dry food
- ✓ **If there are other cats in the house, allow them to have hiding place or "time-out" safe spots.**

DIAGNOSING URINARY TRACT PROBLEMS

Since the signs and symptoms of the various urinary tract problems that affect cats are similar, your veterinarian will need to play detective to uncover the reason for your cat's problems. The first step is a physical examination, during which your veterinarian may discover signs of lower urinary tract disease, such as a thickened or inflamed bladder wall. A variety of tests are needed to help pinpoint the cause. These can include the following:

- **Urine culture,** which can identify the type of bacterial growth. Because the urine sample must be free of any environmental contamination, it is collected using cystocentesis, which involves inserting a needle into the cat's bladder to withdraw the sample. It takes forty-eight hours to get the results of a urine culture.
- **Urine analysis,** which evaluates the urine sample for pH balance and the presence of infection, blood, glucose, and protein levels.
- **X-rays and ultrasound,** which are used to identify any bladder stones and crystals in the urine

Depending on what the veterinarian finds and the cat's health history and symptoms, tests to rule out kidney problems and diabetes also may be done.

CONVENTIONAL TREATMENT

The treatment your veterinarian recommends will depend on the specific problem (e.g., presence of stones or partial or complete blockage of the urethra) and its severity. Cats who have a mild case of feline lower urinary tract disease may be prescribed antibiotics alone. Depending on the cat's symptoms, veterinarians may also prescribe amitriptyline, an antidepressant, as well as a painkiller to help the cat work through the symptoms.

Cats who have stones (crystals) may be given fluid therapy to reduce the concentration of the urine, which in turn cuts down the chances of crystals forming. Fluid therapy is delivered via a catheter, typically placed in a vein in the cat's front leg. A urinary catheter is then placed in the urethra so the crystals can be flushed out.

Some cats do not respond well to the flushing procedure and are not completely cleared, so they need surgery. The procedure is called a perineal urethrostomy, and it involves partially amputating the penis so the urethral opening will be larger. This procedure is successful in most cases, although a small number of cats still experience blockage after surgery.

If your cat is unable to pee at all, this is an emergency situation. In such a case, your veterinarian will need to drain the urine from the bladder, which can be done by placing a syringe into your cat's bladder and withdrawing the urine before performing surgery to open up the blockage. To treat a cat who has a urethral obstruction, a catheter is usually passed up the urethra. After the obstruction has been cleared, the cat will need to be hospitalized for several days, during which time she will be given antibiotics to help prevent infection and other treatments as necessary, such as intravenous fluids or drugs to help restore function of the bladder.

HOME REMEDIES

As a pet parent, there is much you can do to take care of your cat using home remedies for urinary tract problems. At the top of the list is diet, regardless of the type of urinary problem your cat has or the symptoms he is experiencing. Other home remedies can be used along with dietary changes to effectively and safely treat your cat and prevent future episodes of urinary tract problems.

Diet

If you take away only one message from this chapter, please let it be this one: Banish dry cat food from your home. To avoid urinary tract infections and disease, feed your cat canned food and/or a homemade diet. Yes, I know you've heard this recommendation before, but a urinary tract problem is one type of condition that is especially associated with consumption of dry cat food.

Another significant part of your cat's dietary change is water. Although switching to canned food or homemade food from dry cat food is an important change, it's also a good idea to encourage your cat to drink more water. A few little tricks include adding a small amount of additional water to the food, putting a little fluid from canned tuna (packed in water) into the water bowl, and introducing your cat to a feline watering fountain, which stimulates some cats to drink more.

Barley Water

If you have ever simmered barley in water, you likely noticed that the water in which it cooked had a slightly mucous quality. It turns out that this sticky water has healing qualities because it can soothe the mucous membranes and help reduce pain and inflammation.

To prepare barley water for your cat, combine 10 parts water to 1 part pearl barley. Boil the water, add the barley, and then simmer until the barley is soft. You may need to add some extra water as it cooks. When the barley is done, allow it to cool and then strain through cheesecloth or a fine sieve. (Hint: You can enjoy the barley; your cat needs the water.) Give your cat about a teaspoon or two daily for about one week. You may want to make small amounts, as barley water, even when refrigerated, does not keep well past twenty-four hours, so you will need to make new batches daily.

Cranberry

Cranberry has a reputation as being helpful in preventing urinary tract infections in people by stopping bacteria from sticking to the bladder wall, which allows the body to eliminate the bacteria more easily. The same may be true for cats, although there are no scientific studies to back up this idea. However, many of the studies of cranberry and urinary tract infections have been done in lab animals, and they have responded well.

Therefore, if you can get your cat to consume cranberry juice, it may be helpful. Skip the stuff they sell in the supermarket: It's easy to make your own (and keep some for yourself too!). In a large pot containing 4½ cups of water, add 2 cups of ground up fresh or frozen cranberries. Simmer the cranberries on low heat until they are very soft. Remove the mixture from the heat and strain through a fine sieve or cheesecloth. Refrigerate the juice.

The suggested dose of cranberry juice is 1 milliliter per pound of body weight daily, and it should be given for at least seven days, even if the urinary tract infection appears to have been cleared. If Kitty refuses to drink the juice, you can try mixing it with a small amount of yogurt.

Another option is a cranberry supplement. A typical dose is 250 mg of cranberry extract daily, but you should consult your veterinarian before deciding on a dose. Never give cranberry to a cat who has chronic kidney failure, because the fruit contains benzoic acid, which cannot be broken down by cats who have renal failure.

Glucosamine and Chondroitin

Cats do not suffer from arthritis nearly as much as dogs do, but when they do, a natural home remedy is glucosamine and chondroitin. You may even be familiar with these supplements as treatments for arthritis in people. However, both glucosamine and chondroitin, when used together, also can benefit cats who have feline lower urinary tract disease. Supplements of glucosamine can help restore glycosaminoglycans, compounds that are found in the lining of the bladder wall. If you provide chondroitin as well, you can help prevent glycosaminoglycans from being broken down. Therefore, together these supplements can reduce inflammation of the bladder and help resolve symptoms of urinary tract disease. A typical dose is 100 mg of glucosamine per 10 pounds of body weight, while chondroitin is dosed at 50 mg per 10 pounds of body weight.

Parsley Tea

We can probably thank the early settlers of the United States for the use of parsley in the treatment of urinary tract problems. Parsley tea was often used to manage kidney and bladder problems as well as water retention. Your cat can also benefit from this home remedy. Add 1 heaping tablespoon of finely chopped fresh parsley to 8 ounces of boiling water. Remove the water from the heat and steep the parsley for twenty minutes. Strain off the parsley and allow the brew to cool before offering it to your cat. You may need to entice your cat to drink the parsley water by adding a few drops of water from canned tuna (packed in water, not oil). Provide the parsley water daily for one week.

Vitamin C

Adding a vitamin C (as ascorbic acid) to your cat's food may help reduce inflammation and support the integrity of the bladder lining. A typical dose is 250 to 500 mg twice a day, depending on your cat's weight. Consult your veterinarian for the optimal dose for your cat. Vitamin C makes the urine more acidic and also aids in preventing the formation of bladder stones. Some cats experience loose stools when taking vitamin C, but this side effect can be eliminated by lowering the dose.

20+ Things Your Cat Should Avoid

This list was compiled from various veterinary sources. Not every veterinary expert agrees with the presence of every item on this list, so I have included a brief explanation to any entry for which there is some debate.

Alcohol. Your cat is not your drinking buddy. Alcohol can result in coma and death in cats.

Baby food. Your cat may be your baby, but human infant food is not nutritionally suitable for a cat. Some baby foods also contain onion powder, and onions are toxic to cats.

Bones. Raw food advocates do not agree with this no-no, although it can be quantified to say that only raw chicken bones are acceptable, while those from meat sources and fish are not. The objections to bones include risk of contamination (raw bones) plus the risk of splintering and resulting lacerations and obstruction of the digestive system. Cooked bones are softer and therefore much more likely to cause the latter problems than are raw bones.

Caffeine. You may need to get charged up in the morning, but your cat doesn't. Avoid allowing your cat to consume anything that has caffeine in it, including coffee, tea, chocolate, colas, and power drinks. In addition to caffeine, these items also contain theobromine or theophylline, and all of these substances are damaging to the nervous system and the heart, and can also cause diarrhea, vomiting, muscle tremors, rapid breathing, seizures, and restlessness.

Canned tuna. Cats typically love tuna, but tuna canned for human consumption does not have the same nutrients found in tuna prepared for cats. Feeding your cat large amounts of tuna meant for you can result in a thiamine deficiency for your cat.

Dog food. You may have heard the warning about dogs, cats, and their food: Dogs can safely eat cat food, but cats should not eat dog food, because food for dogs does not contain taurine, a nutrient essential for a cat's heart and overall health.

Fat. Cooked or uncooked fat trimmed from meat and poultry should not be given to cats, as it can cause pancreatitis, or inflammation of the pancreas. This is a potentially life-threatening disease.

Liver. But isn't liver in commercial cat food? Yes, but in very small amounts. Cats who eat too much liver can experience vitamin A toxicity, which can damage your cat's bones and, in some cases, cause death.

Macadamia nuts. These delicious nuts contain a substance that is toxic to cats and have negative effects on the muscles and the digestive and nervous systems.

Marijuana. If you partake, it is not cool to allow your cat to do the same. Marijuana can cause vomiting, changes in heart rate, and a suppressed nervous system in cats.

Milk and dairy products. Although kittens tolerate milk, adult cats typically do not and will develop diarrhea and other digestive problems. Avoid giving your cat milk or other products made from milk.

Mushrooms. I'm talking about wild mushrooms that may crop up in your yard or other areas where your cat may roam if he goes outside. Wild mushrooms often contain toxins that can cause seizures, hallucinations, coma, or death.

Onions and garlic. Onions, shallots, and scallions either raw, cooked, or powder are considered dangerous for cats because they contain substances (disulfides, sulfoxides) that can cause anemia. Garlic is less dangerous for cats, and in fact many veterinarians believe that small amounts of garlic, taken for a short time to help manage certain situations such as fleas, are safe. In fact, there are supplements for cats that contain garlic. Other veterinary experts, however, recommend avoiding garlic completely.

Persimmons. I don't know of many cats who have access to persimmons, but if yours does, keep her away. The seeds can obstruct the intestinal tract and cause inflammation (enteritis).

Raisins and grapes. Although these seem like fun treats for cats, they, along with currants, contain an unknown toxin that can cause kidney damage.

Raw food. Raw food advocates will not agree with this entry, but there are two sides to the raw food story. Raw eggs, for example, may contain salmonella, which can result in food poisoning. They also contain avidin, an enzyme that reduces the ability of the body to absorb biotin, which can result in skin and hair coat problems. Raw meat, poultry, and fish also can contain harmful bacteria, such as E. coli, campylobacter, vibrio, salmonella, and listeria, as well as parasites. Pet parents who choose to give their cats a raw food diet may help reduce these risks by purchasing organically raised meat, poultry, fish, and eggs.

Rhubarb leaves. Unless you have a garden or your cat has access to rhubarb growing somewhere, the chances he will chew on rhubarb leaves is unlikely. However, these leaves contain oxalates, which can cause problems with the nervous, digestive, and urinary systems.

Salt. Hold the saltshaker! Small amounts of salt are safe, but too much can cause an imbalance of electrolytes in your cat.

Yeast dough. If you like to bake, make sure kitty isn't hanging around to sample the yeast dough. Munching on the dough can cause accumulation of gas in her digestive tract, and even result in a ruptured stomach or intestines.

Endnotes

Chapter 1

Kirk, Claudia, quote re calcium, from Medicine.net: http://
www.medicinenet.com/pets/dog-health/homemade_dog
_food-page2.htm.

Hewson-Hughes AK et al. Geometric analysis of macronutrient selection in the adult domestic cat, *Felis catus. Journal
of Experimental Biology* 2011 Mar 15; 214:1039–51.

Chapter 2

Petfoodtalk.com: http://petfoodtalk.com/catfoodreviews/.

AAFCO Nutritional List for Cat from *Merck Manual*: http://
www.merckvetmanual.com/mvm/htm/bc/tmgn47.htm.

Chapter 3

Consumer Media Network: The Raw Facts: Dog Diets. Accessed Sept. 3, 2012. http://www.cmn.com/2012/03/the
-raw-facts-dog-diets/.

Kerr KR et al. Apparent total tract energy and macronutrient digestibility and fecal fermentative end-product concentrations of domestic cats fed extruded, raw beef-based,
and cooked beef-based diets. *Journal of Animal Science*
2012; 90:515–22.

Schlesinger DP, Joffe DJ. Raw food diets in companion animals: a critical review. *Canadian Veterinary Journal*
2011 Jan; 52(1): 50–54.

Chapter 4

Ganz EC et al. Evaluation of methylprednisolone and triamcinolone for the induction and maintenance treatment of pruritus in allergic cats: a double-blinded, randomized, prospective study. *Veterinary Dermatology* 2012, Oct; 23(5): 387

Griffin JS et al. An open clinical trial on the efficacy of cetirizine hydrochloride in the management of allergic pruritus in cats. *Canadian Veterinary Journal* 2012 Jan; 53(1): 47–50.

Heinrich NA et al. Adverse events in 50 cats with allergic dermatitis receiving ciclosporin. *Veterinary Dermatology* 2011 Dec; 22(6): 511–20.

Chapter 5

Araujo JA et al. Tablets improve executive function in aged dogs and cats: implications for treatment of cognitive dysfunction syndrome. *International Journal of Applied Research in Veterinary Medicine* 2012; 10(1): 90–98.

Bain, Melissa, DVM, DACVB. Cognitive dysfunction in older cats. Best Friends. Accessed August 3, 2012. http://www.bestfriends.org/theanimals/pdfs/cats/catcognitivedysfunction.pdf.

Dowling AL, Head E. Antioxidants in the canine model of human aging. *Biochim Biophys Acta* 2012 May; 1822(50): 685–89.

Gunn-Moore D. Apparent senility in geriatric cats. Accessed August 3, 2012. http://www.fabcats.org/owners/elderly/senility.html.

Gunn-Moore DA. Cognitive dysfunction in cats: clinical assessment and management. *Top Companion Animal Medicine* 2011 Feb; 26(1): 17–24.

Head E et al. Effects of age, dietary, and behavioral enrichment on brain mitochondria in a canine model of human aging. *Experimental Neurology* 2009 Nov; 220(1): 171–76.

Landsberg GM et al. Cognitive dysfunction in cats: a syndrome we used to dismiss as "old age." *Journal of Feline Medicine and Surgery* 2010 Nov; 12(11): 837–48.

Milgram NW et al. Acetyl-L-carnitine and alpha-lipoic acid supplementation of aged beagle dogs improves learning in two landmark discrimination tests. *FASEB Journal* 2007 Nov; 21(13): 3756–62.

Reme CA et al. Effect of S-adenosylmethionine tablets on the reduction of age-related mental decline in dogs: a double-blinded, placebo-controlled trial. *Veterinary Therapy* 2008 Summer; 9(2): 69–82.

VetInfo.com. http://www.vetinfo.com/category/cats/.

Chapter 6

Hudson JB. Applications of the phytomedicine echinacea purpurea (purple coneflower) in infectious diseases. *Journal of Biomedicine & Biotechnology* 2012; 2012: 769896.

Kawabata F, Tsuji T. Effects of dietary supplementation with a combination of fish oil, bilberry extract, and lutein on subjective symptoms of asthenopia in humans. *Biomedical Research* 2011 Dec; 32(6): 387–93.

Matsunaga N et al. Bilberry and its main constituents have neuroprotective effects against retinal neuronal damage in vitro and in vivo. *Molecular Nutritional Food Research* 2009 Jul; 53(7): 869–77.

Chapter 7

Hodgkins, Elizabeth H. *Your Cat: Simple New Secrets to a Longer, Stronger Life*. New York: St. Martin's, 2007.

Chapter 8

Appleton DJ et al. Dietary chromium tripicolinate supplementation reduces glucose concentrations and improves glucose tolerance in normal-weight cats. *Journal of Feline Medicine and Surgery* 2002 Mar; 4(1): 13–25.

Elliott D. Quoted in "Most common dog, cat diseases revealed." From Discovery.com May 19, 2011. http://news.discovery.com/animals/pets-health-cats-dogs-110519.html.

Hoenig M. The cat as a model for human obesity and diabetes. *Journal of Diabetes and Science Technology* 2012 May 1; 6(3): 525–33.

Mazzaferro EM et al. Treatment of feline diabetes mellitus using an alpha-glucosidase inhibitor and a low-carbohydrate diet. *Journal of Feline Medicine and Surgery* 2003 Jun; 5(3): 183–89.

Nelson RW, DVM. From WebMD: http://pets.webmd.com/cats/guide/feeding-tips-for-a-cat-with-diabetes.

Rand JS et al. Diet in the prevention of diabetes and obesity in companion animals. *Asia Pacific Journal of Clinical Nutrition* 2003; 12 Suppl S6.

Smith JR et al. A survey of southeastern United States veterinarians' preferences of managing cats with diabetes mellitus. *Journal of Feline Medicine & Surgery* 2012 Oct; 14(10): 716–22

YourDiabeticCat.com. Accessed July 26, 2012. http://yourdiabeticcat.com/index.html.

State of Pet Health 2011 Report: http://news.discovery.com/animals/pets-health-cats-dogs-110519.html.

Chapter 10

Associated Press. Quotes from "Ohio State studies symptoms of cat stress, disease" by Sue Manning, Jan. 10, 2011.

The Conscious Cat. Minimizing stress for cats can decrease illness. http://consciouscat.net/2011/01/24/minimizing-stress-for-cats-can-decrease-illnes/.

Westropp JL et al. Evaluation of the effects of stress in cats with idiopathic cystitis. *American Journal of Veterinary Research* 2006 Apr; 67(4): 731–36.

Chapter 12

Dann JR et al. A potential nutritional prophylactic for the reduction of feline hairball symptoms. *The Journal of Nutrition* 2004 Aug 1; 134(8): 21245–55.

Chapter 13

Benvenga S et al. Usefulness of L-carnitine, a naturally occurring peripheral antagonist of thyroid hormone action, in iatrogenic hyperthyroidism: a randomized double blind, placebo-controlled clinical trial. *Journal of Clinical Endocrinology & Metabolism* 2001 Aug; 86(8): 3579–94.

Dye JA et al. Elevated PBDE levels in pet cats: sentinels for humans? *Environmental Science & Technology* 2007 Sep 15; 41(18): 6350–56.

Edinboro CH et al. Feline hyperthyroidism: potential relationship with iodine supplement requirements of commercial cat foods. *Journal of Feline Medical Surgery* 2010 Sep; 12(9): 672–79.

Feline Advisory Board (FAB). www.fabcats.org

Frenais R et al. Clinical efficacy and safety of a once-daily formulation of carbimazole in cats with hyperthyroidism. *Journal of Small Animal Practice* 2009 Oct; 50 (10): 510–15.

Hill KE et al. The efficacy and safety of a novel lipophilic formulation of methimazole for the once daily transdermal treatment of cats with hyperthyroidism. *Journal of Veterinary Internal Medicine* 2011 Nov–Dec; 25(6): 1357–65.

Chapter 14

AnniesRemedy.com. Kitchen Medicine. http://www.annies remedy.com/chart_remedy.php?rem_ID=468.

Guerrini VH, Kriticos CM. Effects of azadirachtin on Ctenocephalides feis in the dog and the cat. *Veterinary Parasitology* 1998 Jan 31; 74(2–4): 289–97.

Lans C et al. Ethnoveterinary medicines used to treat endo-
parasites and stomach problems in pigs and pets in Brit-
ish Columbia, Canada. *Veterinary Parasitology* 2007 Sep
30; 148(3–4): 325–40.

Pitcairn, Richard H, DVM. *Dr. Pitcairn's New Complete
Guide to Natural Health for Dogs and Cats*. Emmaus,
PA: Rodale, 2005.

Travers MA et al. Probiotics for the control of parasites:
an overview. *Journal of Parasitology Research* 201;
2011:610769.

Chapter 15

Hodgkins, Elizabeth M. *Your Cat: Simple New Secrets to a
Longer, Stronger Life*. New York: St. Martin's, 2007, pp.
211–27.

Kidder AC, Chew D. Treatment options for hyperphosphate-
mia in feline CKD: what's out there? *Journal of Feline
Medicine & Surgery* 2009 Nov; 11(11): 913–24.

Chapter 16

Association for Pet Obesity Prevention study 2011:
http://www.petmd.com/news/health-science/nws_multi_US
_pets_obese_too#.UClD47QV3Xs.

Barry, D. Catnip: The key chemical responsible for the
herb's frisk-inducing effects on felines is nepetalactone.
Chemical & Engineering News 2005 Aug; 83(13): 39.

Center SA et al. The clinical and metabolic effects of rapid
weight loss in obese pet cats and the influence of supplemental oral L-carnitine. *Journal of Veterinary Internal
Medicine* 200 Nov–Dec; 14(6): 598–608.

Pierson, Lisa DVM. http://www.catinfo.org/?link=feline
obesity#Is_Your_Cat_Overweight.

Chapter 17

Litster A et al. Feline bacterial urinary tract infections: an update on an evolving clinical problem. *Veterinary Journal* 2011 Jan; 187(1): 18–22.

Weese JS et al. Antimicrobial use guidelines for treatment of urinary tract disease in dogs and cats: antimicrobial guidelines working group of the international society for companion animal infectious diseases. *Veterinary Medicine International* 2011; 2011:263768.

Suggested Reading/Sources

Alinovi, Cathy, CVM, and Susan Thixton. *Dinner PAWsible: A Cookbook for Healthy Nutritious Meals for Cats and Dogs.* CreateSpace, 2011.

Fox, Michael W., BVet, PhD., et al. *Not Fit For a Dog: The Truth about Manufactured Cat & Dog Food.* Scottsdale, AZ: Linder Publishing, 2012.

Frazier, Anitra. *The Natural Cat: The Comprehensive Guide to Optimum Care.* London: Quarry Books, 2006.

Hodgkins, Elizabeth M., DVM, Esq. *Your Cat: Simple New Secrets to a Longer, Stronger Life.* New York: St. Martin's, 2007.

Kahn, Cynthia M., ed. *The Merck/Merial Manual for Pet Health: The Complete Pet Health Resource for Your Dog, Cat, Horse, or Other Pets—in Everyday Language.* Whitehouse Station, NJ: Merck & Co., 2007.

Martin, Ann N., and Shawn Messonnier. *Food Pets Die For: Shocking Facts about Pet Food,* 3rd ed. Trootdale, OR: New Sage Press, 2008.

Messonnier, Shawn, DVM. *Natural Health Bible for Dogs & Cats: Your A–Z Guide to Over 200 Conditions, Herb, Vitamins, and Supplements.* New York: Three Rivers Press, 2001.

Nestle, Marion. *Pet Food Politics: The Chihuahua in the Coal Mine.* Berkeley: University of California Press, 2010.

Nestle, Marion, and Malden Nesheim. *Feed Your Pet Right: The Authoritative Guide to Feeding Your Dog and Cat.* New York: Free Press, 2010.

Pitcairn, Richard H., and Susan H. Pitcairn. *Dr. Pitcairn's New Complete Guide to Natural Health for Dogs and Cats.* Emmaus, PA: Rodale, 2005.

Schenck, Patricia, DVM. *Home-Prepared Dog & Cat Diets,* 2nd ed. Hoboken, NJ: Blackwell Publishing, 2010.

Shiroff, Lisa. *Purr-fect Recipes for a Healthy Cat: 101 Natural Cat Food and Treat Recipes to Make Your Cat Happy.* Ocala, FL: Atlantic Publishing, 2011.

Straw, D. *Why Is Cancer Killing Our Pets?* Rochester, VT: Healing Arts Press, 2000.

Yarnall, Celeste, DVM, and Hofue, Jean. *The Complete Guide to Holistic Cat Care.* London: Quarry Books, 2009.

Sources of Information on Feline Health and Cat Food

The following is a representative list only and is no way an endorsement of any company or organization.

Association for Pet Obesity Prevention (APOP)
http://www.petobesityprevention.com/pet-weight-translator/
This association provides highly informative and comprehensive information on obesity prevention and treatment.

Cat Health
http://www.cathealth.com/
Articles on cat health, grooming, toys, cat care, and other feline topics.

Catinfo.org
http://www.catinfo.org/
Provides comprehensive, critical information on how to take care of your cat, especially regarding diet, by a feline specialist, Lisa A. Pierson, DVM.

ConsumerLab.com
http://www.consumerlab.com/
Provides reviews of a wide range of supplements. Primarily a site for human supplements, but it does have some pet products. Only some information is free; there is a subscription price as well.

Cornell University Feline Health Center
http://www.vet.cornell.edu/fhc/hinformation.htm
Information for pet parents and veterinarians on cat health.

Feline Advisory Board
http://www.fabcats.org/
The Feline Advisory Board runs a Web site called Fabcats, which provides information on health and welfare issues concerning cats. Although this charity is headquartered in the United Kingdom, caring about cats is universal, and the information crosses all borders.

National Animal Supplement Council
http://nasc.cc/
An organization whose members are manufacturers of animal health supplements and who strive to improve the quality of these products sold for cats, dogs, and other companion animals.

Truth About Pet Food
http://www.truthaboutpetfood.com/
A thorough, comprehensive source of information about pet food, including articles, reviews, tips, recall information, industry news, pet food regulations, and more.

Veterinary Information
http://www.vetinfo.com/
Scores of articles on cat health by veterinarians and other experts.